FREE Study Skills DVD O...

Dear Customer,

Thank you for your purchase from Mometrix! We consider it an honor and privilege that you have purchased our product and want to ensure your satisfaction.

As a way of showing our appreciation and to help us better serve you, we have developed a Study Skills DVD that we would like to give you for <u>FREE</u>. **This DVD covers our "best practices" for studying for your exam, from using our study materials to preparing for the day of the test.**

All that we ask is that you email us your feedback that would describe your experience so far with our product. Good, bad or indifferent, we want to know what you think!

To get your **FREE Study Skills DVD**, email <u>freedvd@mometrix.com</u> with "FREE STUDY SKILLS DVD" in the subject line and the following information in the body of the email:

    a. The name of the product you purchased.

    b. Your product rating on a scale of 1-5, with 5 being the highest rating.

    c. Your feedback. It can be long, short, or anything in-between, just your impressions and experience so far with our product. Good feedback might include how our study material met your needs and will highlight features of the product that you found helpful.

    d. Your full name and shipping address where you would like us to send your free DVD.

If you have any questions or concerns, please don't hesitate to contact me directly.

Thanks again!

Sincerely,

Jay Willis
Vice President
<u>jay.willis@mometrix.com</u>
1-800-673-8175

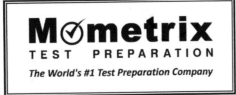

ATI TEAS®
Practice Questions

Two TEAS 6 Practice Tests & Review for the
Test of Essential Academic Skills, Sixth Edition

Published by
Mometrix Test Preparation
TEAS Exam Secrets Test Prep Team

Written and edited by the TEAS Exam Secrets Test Prep Staff

Printed in the United States of America

This paper meets the requirements of ANSI/NISO Z39.48-1992 (Permanence of Paper).

Mometrix offers volume discount pricing to institutions. For more information or a price quote, please contact our sales department at sales@mometrix.com or 888-248-1219.

ATI TEAS® is a registered trademark of the Assessment Technologies Institute ®, which was not involved in the production of, and does not endorse, this product.

ISBN 13: 978-1-5167-0692-1
ISBN 10: 1-5167-0692-7

Table of Contents

TEAS Practice Test #1

Reading

DIRECTIONS: The reading practice test you are about to take is multiple-choice with only one correct answer per question. Read each test item and circle your answer on the answer sheet below. When you have completed the practice test, you may check your answers with the answers on the answer key following the test.

Answer Sheet

1.	a	b	c	d		28.	a	b	c	d
2.	a	b	c	d		29.	a	b	c	d
3.	a	b	c	d		30.	a	b	c	d
4.	a	b	c	d		31.	a	b	c	d
5.	a	b	c	d		32.	a	b	c	d
6.	a	b	c	d		33.	a	b	c	d
7.	a	b	c	d		34.	a	b	c	d
8.	a	b	c	d		35.	a	b	c	d
9.	a	b	c	d		36.	a	b	c	d
10.	a	b	c	d		37.	a	b	c	d
11.	a	b	c	d		38.	a	b	c	d
12.	a	b	c	d		39.	a	b	c	d
13.	a	b	c	d		40.	a	b	c	d
14.	a	b	c	d		41.	a	b	c	d
15.	a	b	c	d		42.	a	b	c	d
16.	a	b	c	d		43.	a	b	c	d
17.	a	b	c	d		44.	a	b	c	d
18.	a	b	c	d		45.	a	b	c	d
19.	a	b	c	d		46.	a	b	c	d
20.	a	b	c	d		47.	a	b	c	d
21.	a	b	c	d		48.	a	b	c	d
22.	a	b	c	d		49.	a	b	c	d
23.	a	b	c	d		50.	a	b	c	d
24.	a	b	c	d		51.	a	b	c	d
25.	a	b	c	d		52.	a	b	c	d
26.	a	b	c	d		53.	a	b	c	d
27.	a	b	c	d						

The next two questions are based on the following passage.

In the American Southwest of the late 1800s, the introduction of barbed wire fencing led to fierce disputes between ranchers and farmers, both eager to protect their rights and their livelihood. The farmers were the clear winners of the two groups, and the barbed wire fences stayed and proliferated. Barbed wire proved to be ideal for use in western conditions; it was cheaper and easier to use than the alternatives of wood fences, stone walls or hedges. Within a few decades all the previously open range land became fenced-in private property. This change was so dramatic to the western culture that some consider the introduction of barbed wire fencing to be the event that ended the Old West period of our history.

1. Which of the following did the author <u>not</u> mention would have been found in the Old West prior to the introduction of barbed wire fencing?
    a. wood fences
    b. hedges
    c. stone walls
    d. none of the above

2. According to the author, when did the introduction of barbed wire fencing occur?
    a. the late 16th century
    b. the late 17th century
    c. the late 18th century
    d. the late 19th century

3. If an author argues that children like strawberries more than any other fruit, what would be the best evidence to support her argument?
    a. A diary written by one child
    b. An interview from a kindergarten teacher
    c. An article about strawberries from a school paper
    d. A survey of 500 children that supports the author's theory

4. The text feature of **boldface** is most often used to indicate which of these?
    a. A word that has a footnote at the page bottom
    b. A word that is listed and defined in the glossary
    c. The words of the captions accompanying visuals
    d. The words of all text in sidebars on some pages

5. Of the following, which expression that could be found in informational text uses words in a figurative sense rather than a literal one?
    a. An onslaught of criticism
    b. An avalanche of rumors
    c. A throng of onlookers
    d. A belligerent mob

The next three questions are based on the following passage.

This formula is for people with deficiencies and anemic conditions. It aids in the body's absorption of vital minerals such as iron, calcium, zinc, potassium, and sulfur. Take the following ingredients:

Parsley root   Comfrey root
Yellow dock   Watercress
Nettles   Kelp
Irish moss

Slowly simmer equal parts of these herbs with four ounces to a half-quart of water. Continue to simmer slowly until the volume of liquid is reduced by half. Strain, reserve the liquid, and cover the herbs with water once more. Then simmer again for 10 minutes. Strain and combine the two liquids. Cook the liquid down until the volume is reduced by half. Add an equal amount of blackstrap molasses. Take one tablespoon two to four times daily, not exceeding four tablespoons in a 24-hour period.

6. What is the main reason for taking this formula?
    a. to serve as a mineral supplement
    b. to get rid of unnecessary minerals
    c. to reduce the absorption of minerals
    d. to increase the absorption of minerals

7. If a $\frac{1}{4}$ ounce of yellow dock is used, how much watercress should be used?
    a. $\frac{1}{2}$ ounce
    b. $\frac{1}{4}$ ounce
    c. $\frac{1}{3}$ ounce
    d. 1 ounce

8. If a patient follows the directions correctly, how often could the medicine be taken?
    a. once every two hours
    b. once every four hours
    c. once every three hours
    d. once every six hours

---

9. A high school class reads an essay about the possible effects of sexual activity on teens. The author's position is very clear: She believes young people should avoid sex because they aren't mature enough to take the necessary steps to remain safe. The author cites facts, research studies, and statistics to strengthen her position. This type of writing is called:
    a. Expository
    b. Narrative
    c. Persuasive
    d. Didactic

10. Which of the following statements represents the BEST way to evaluate the information in a source?
    a. Make an educated guess about the source's accuracy.
    b. Assume any printed source is completely accurate.
    c. Get in touch with the person who wrote the source.
    d. Check it against information in one or more other sources.

11. Among figures of speech, which of the following is a simile?
    a. Having butterflies in the stomach
    b. Climbing up the ladder of success
    c. Something being light as a feather
    d. Someone having hit a sales target

The next question is based on the following passage.

What Are the Key Facts about Seasonal Flu Vaccine?
Center for Disease Control and Prevention (CDC)

The single best way to protect against the flu is to get vaccinated each year.

About 2 weeks after vaccination, antibodies that provide protection against influenza virus infection develop in the body.

Yearly flu vaccination should begin in September or as soon as vaccine is available and continue throughout the influenza season, into December, January, and beyond. This is because the timing and duration of influenza seasons vary. While influenza outbreaks can happen as early as October, most of the time influenza activity peaks in January or later.

In general, anyone who wants to reduce their chances of getting the flu can get vaccinated. However, it is recommended by ACIP that certain people should get vaccinated each year. They are either people who are at high risk of having serious flu complications or people who live with or care for those at high risk for serious complications. During flu seasons when vaccine supplies are limited or delayed, ACIP makes recommendations regarding priority groups for vaccination.

People who should get vaccinated each year are:
- Children aged 6 months up to their 19th birthday

- 4 -

- Pregnant women
- People 50 years of age and older
- People of any age with certain chronic medical conditions
- People who live in nursing homes and other long-term care facilities
- People who live with or care for those at high risk for complications from flu, including:
  - Health care workers
  - Household contacts of persons at high risk for complications from the flu
  - Household contacts and out of home caregivers of children less than 6 months of age (these children are too young to be vaccinated)

12. Which of the following is a valid summary of the selection?
    a. Older people are especially at risk for the flu.
    b. Flu vaccines should be distributed to all without cost.
    c. People need flu shots in September or it's too late.
    d. Getting an annual flu vaccine is a key step in maintaining good health.

13. Which common mode of writing is most characterized by the author's assumption that certain things are facts or truths?
    a. Informative
    b. Descriptive
    c. Persuasive
    d. Narrative

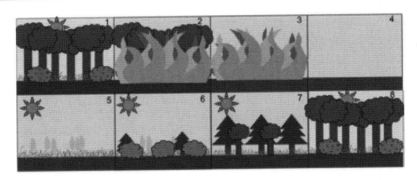

14. This figure shows the ecological succession of vegetation in a temperate deciduous forest after a natural disaster such as a forest fire. Based on the figure above, which of the following is the BEST description of ecological succession?
    a. Succession is a rapid process, and all stages of development occur simultaneously.
    b. Succession is a rapid, ordered progression.
    c. Succession is a gradual, ordered progression.
    d. Succession is a gradual, random process.

The next three questions are based on the following passage.

What's Real About It?

I suppose I don't understand why it is called reality television. It has been argued that reality television has been a part of television since the beginnings of television programming. Through game shows and daytime talk shows, real people, as in non-actors, have made appearances on television for the entertainment of others. A new genre of reality television that became the new phenomenon, however, was introduced in the year 2000, with shows such as "Survivor."

The idea behind "Survivor" is like many in reality television. There are contestants, they are put in extreme situations, and in the end, someone wins a prize. The other main style of reality television involves cameras following someone around as they live their daily life.

My confusion comes from the title of reality. Reality means the state of which things actually exist, but reality television does not display the state in which life actually exists. In real life, not many people will be deserted on a distant island or forced to live in a house with several strangers. Additionally, cameras do not follow people around on a normal day. People live their lives, and exist in a reality that is not meant for entertainment or for masses of people to watch.

It is no surprise to discover that most audiences find it interesting to watch people who are not actors on television. There is something intriguing about fame for the average person. It is as if the viewer can relate more to the show that he or she is watching, because it is real people put in fake situations rather than fake people and characters acting in life-like situations. However, there cannot be anything called reality television that would be both an accurate description of life and provide necessary entertainment.

15. What is the main argument of this essay?
    a. Reality television is not entertainment
    b. Reality television uses actors
    c. The basis of reality television is not reality
    d. Most people do not enjoy reality television

16. Which of the following statements is not an opinion?
    a. "Reality means the state of which things actually exist"
    b. "There is something intriguing about fame for the average person"
    c. "I suppose I don't understand why it is called reality television"
    d. "It is as if the viewer can relate more to the show that he or she is watching"

17. Why does the author assume audiences like to watch reality television?
    a. They enjoy watching real-life situations
    b. Viewers can relate more to real people than actors
    c. They wish they could be celebrities
    d. They want to win prizes

18. Which of the following choices would be most essential to an argument in favor of global environmental protection?
   a. a personal story about how you have witnessed the destruction of the environment in your own neighborhood
   b. a newspaper editorial about illegal garbage dumping
   c. a photograph of a rain forest damaged by pollution
   d. scientifically supported statistics detailing how pollution has damaged the environment throughout the world

---

Power Fruit
"All natural fruit juice that gives you energy all day long!"

35 mg of caffeine
50% daily value of Vitamin E
100% daily value of Vitamin C

19. The advertisement above shows the nutrition information for the new juice, "Power Fruit". Which conclusion can be made about Power Fruit?
   a. Power Fruit contains the daily value of caffeine
   b. Power Fruit provides all the vitamin C you need each day
   c. Power Fruit has 100% daily value of vitamin A
   d. Power Fruit does not contain iron

The next four questions are based on the following ad.

City of Elm Babysitting/ Nanny Jobs Wanted	
College sophomore, aged 20, seeks regular part-time nanny work. Weekends (Sat and Sun) only. Up to three kids, any age range. Have four years of babysitting experience. References available. Contact Lisa, 634-1966.	Very responsible and reliable high-school junior available for occasional babysitting. I love kids and they love me! Personal references available. Contact Jose at 422-6868.
Experienced nanny seeks full-time (M-F, 9-5) nanny position. Over 10 years' experience as nanny. Many, including local, references available. Will also consider light housework, cooking. Contact James. 212-1736.	Devoted, experienced, reliable nanny seeks part-time (Tuesday and Thursday) nanny work. Also available for occasional evening and weekend childcare. Contact Regina at 530-1227.

20. If the Malbec family is looking for occasional weekend childcare, which of the people seeking work should they contact?
   a. Lisa and James
   b. Jose and James
   c. James and Regina
   d. Lisa and Regina

21. If the Sulinus need a two-day-a-week babysitter for their four kids, which of the people seeking work is their best choice to contact?
   a. Lisa
   b. Jose
   c. James
   d. Regina

22. According to the ads, which of the people seeking work might also cook dinners for the Canterruni family if that person was hired for childcare?
   a. Lisa
   b. Jose
   c. James
   d. Regina

23. Which of the people seeking work can one infer from the ads is the youngest?
   a. Lisa
   b. Jose
   c. James
   d Regina

---

24. Which of the following words has a positive connotation?
   a. crash
   b. employ
   c. bribe
   d. chic

The next two questions are based on the following passage.

Helen Keller was born on June 27, 1880. She was a happy and healthy child until the age of 19 months when she fell ill with a terrible fever. Although Helen recovered from the fever, it left her both deaf and blind.

Helen was loved and cared for by her doting parents, but her behavior became erratic after she lost her hearing and sight, with unpredictable outbursts of temper. Her parents were at a loss how to reach her and teach her how to behave. Helen herself was frustrated and lonely in her dark, silent world. All of that began to change in March 1887 when Anne Sullivan came to live with the Kellers and be Helen's teacher.

Anne taught Helen to communicate by forming letters with her fingers held in another person's hand. In this way, Teacher, as Helen called her, taught her pupil to spell cake, doll, and milk. However, it was not until Anne spelled w-a-t-e-r in Helen's hands as cold water gushed over both of them that Helen made the exciting connection between the words and the world around her. This connection engendered an insatiable curiosity within Helen. After that day, Helen learned at an incredible rate with Teacher by her side.

Helen went on to graduate from Radcliffe College. She became a famous writer, speaker, and advocate. The story of Helen's remarkable life is known worldwide. Anne Sullivan and Helen Keller were inseparable until Anne's death in 1936. Teacher shined a light in Helen's dark world and showed her the way.

25. What is the author's primary purpose in writing this passage?
    a. To inform people about Helen Keller's college career
    b. To inform people about Anne Sullivan's life
    c. To inform people about services available for the deaf and blind
    d. To inform people about Helen Keller's life

26. What is the author's tone in this passage?
    a. Indifferent
    b. Censorious
    c. Admiring
    d. Impartial

27. Which of the following would best support the idea that "fracking," shooting water and chemicals into the ground at a high pressure to gain access to underground gas stores, may be hazardous to the environment?
    a. a letter in the science journal *Climatic Change* that includes results from research on fracking showing that it may be more damaging to the environment than burning coal
    b. a letter to the editor of the *Chicago Tribune* from an activist who secretly taped what was going on at fracking locations throughout the US
    c. a feature-length movie developed by a former politician that uses special effects to highlight the effects of fracking on climate change
    d. an article in a newspaper discussing the impact of fracking on the local community, noting that all of the people interviewed were nervous about the issue

28. Your teacher has assigned you a research project on ancient Persian culture. Which of the following sources would be a good starting point that provides the most accurate information?
    a. the Wikipedia "Persian Culture" entry
    b. "All Cool Persian Stuff": a blog written by a scientist
    c. *An Overview of Persian Society*: a book written by a historian
    d. "Uncovering the Secrets of Persia": a two-page magazine article about lost temples

In a debate, the first speaker claims that "Students should be allowed to graduate from school after completing the 10th grade, instead of making them attend until they are 18. Most students will not go to college, so it doesn't make sense to waste their time preparing for something that won't happen. These students need the extra years to start working regular jobs and supporting their families. "

29. What might be one counterclaim to this? Choose the answer that provides a counterclaim and evaluates the speaker's argument.
   a. It's silly to say that students don't need to be in school until 18. A person who makes a claim like that has little understanding of the educational system and very little knowledge of real life. While it might be good to start working earlier than 18, who's to say that a student can get a good job?
   b. It is certainly true that most students will never attend college. Statistics show that the majority of high school students fail to show an interest in college. There are also a high number of students who are pushed into going to college that fail the first year because they went for the wrong reasons.
   c. What does a 16-year-old know about life? At 16, you live in your parents' home and are considered a child. If a student drops out at 16, there may be regrets later in life. After all, it is a proven fact that college graduates make considerably more money than workers with less education.
   d. While it is true that most students do not go to college, and that working is beneficial, attending school until 18 is valuable. At 16, most students do not really know what they want to do: if they drop out of school early, they may regret that they lost the chance to study hard and attend college. Research shows that college grads make more money than those with less education.

The next four questions are based on the following radio schedule.

Sunday May 17	
Overnight	
12 a.m.	News from the BBC World headlines from BBC London.
1 a.m.	California Update Upcoming election discussed.
2 a.m.	Money Matters How to protect your retirement if you lose your job.
3 a.m.	Commonwealth Club The Green Economy. Host Stephen Sanders speaks with Nancy Sparks, leading proponent of the idea that green jobs can save the world economy.
4 a.m.	News from the BBC World headlines from BBC London.
5 a.m.	All About Art Host Guy Phillips speaks to three local graffiti artists.
Morning	
7 a.m.	California Update Upcoming election discussed.
9 a.m.	Smart Talk Call-in show about President Obama's first 100 days in office.
10 a.m.	Car Talk Tom & Ray Magliozzi host a call-in show about your car problems.
11 a.m.	Prairie Home Companion Garrison Keillor.

30. What show features talk about an upcoming election?
    a. News from the BBC
    b. California Update
    c. Commonwealth Club
    d. Smart Talk

31. From the information given, on which show would you expect to hear the most discussion about national U.S. politics?
    a. News from the BBC
    b. California Update
    c. Smart Talk
    d. Commonwealth Club

32. On which show would you expect to hear the environment discussed the most?
    a. Prairie Home Companion
    b. Commonwealth Club
    c. California Update
    d. News from the BBC

33. On which show would you be most likely to hear the following "should drawing on someone else's property without their consent be treated as a crime?"
    a. California Report
    b. Car Talk
    c. Commonwealth Club
    d. All About Art

The next three questions are based on the following passage.

On April 30, 1803, the United States bought the Louisiana Territory from the French. Astounded and excited by the offer of a sale and all that it would mean, it took less than a month to hear the offer and determine to buy it for $15 million. Right away the United States had more than twice the amount of land as before, giving the country more of a chance to become powerful. They had to move in military and governmental power in this region, but even as this was happening they had very little knowledge about the area. They did not even really know where the land boundaries were, nor did they have any how many people lived there. They needed to explore.

34. Based on the facts in the passage, what prediction could you make about the time immediately following the Louisiana Purchase?
    a. Explorers were already on the way to the region.
    b. The government wanted to become powerful.
    c. People in government would make sure explorers went to the region.
    d. Explorers would want to be paid for their work.

35. Why did the United States decide to buy the Louisiana Territory?
    a. They wanted to be more powerful.
    b. They wanted to find out the land boundaries.
    c. They wanted to know how many people lived there.
    d. They were astounded.

36. The author writes that "astounded and excited by the offer of a sale and all that it would mean ..." Which of the following words is most synonymous with the word "astounded" as used in that sentence?
    a. eager
    b. confused
    c. greedy
    d. shocked

The next four questions are based on the following table.

Information on Hiking Trails in the Area			
Trail	**Length**	**Level of Difficulty**	**Attractions**
1. Beaverton Falls	2.6 miles	Easy	Three waterfalls with picnic areas open May-September; trail is suitable for all ages. End of trail connects to Copper Creek Trail.
2. Silver Bullet	5.5 miles	Easy – Moderate	Follows the Salmon River; fishing allowed July-October. Meets the Toulanne River and connects to the Toulanne Trail.
3. Eagle Eye	8.2 miles	Moderate – Hard	Trail has steep terrain, narrow segments, and switchbacks. Features two waterfalls and excellent panoramic views at the ridge
4. Toulanne	7.5 miles	Moderate	Beautiful rock formations along trail, with close views of canyon walls and Toulanne River. Boat rentals April-November
5. Copper Creek	9.5 miles	Hard	Icy in winter, and many areas require climbing gear. Caving and climbing gear rentals available year-round.

37. Which trail does not connect to another trail?
    a. Beaverton Falls
    b. Silver Bullet
    c. Eagle Eye
    d. Copper Creek

38. This summer the Esperanza family is planning to have their family reunion outdoors surrounded by beautiful scenery. People of all ages are expected to attend. Which trail would be best for them to use?
    a. Beaverton Falls
    b. Eagle Eye
    c. Toulanne
    d. Copper Creek

39. The Cornell family wants to do some fishing in June. Which trail should they choose?
    a. Beaverton Falls
    b. Eagle Eye
    c. Copper Creek
    d. Toulanne

40. If Joey and Katrina hike an average of 3 miles per hour, about how long will it take them if they take the Beaverton Falls trail and follow it through the Copper Creek trail?
   a. 3 hours
   b. $3\frac{1}{2}$ hours
   c. 4 hours
   d. $4\frac{1}{2}$ hours

41. Follow the numbered instructions to transform the starting word into a different word.
      1. Start with the word MELIORATE.
      2. Remove the letter E from the end of the word.
      3. Remove the letter E from the middle of the word.
      4. Remove the letter L from the middle of the word.
      5. Remove the letter I from the middle of the word.
      6. Add the letter A to the beginning of the word.
      7. Replace the letter T with the letter L.

What new word has been spelled?
   a. amerce
   b. amoral
   c. amenity
   d. melody

42. The guide words at the top of a dictionary page are *degressive* and *delectation*. Which of the following words is an entry on this page?
   a. delegacy
   b. degrade
   c. deject
   d. delirium

43. Which mode of writing is most suitable for the purpose of encouraging the reading audience to explore ideas and consider various potential associated responses?
   a. Narrative
   b. Expository
   c. Persuasive
   d. Speculative

44. Calvin's <u>mordant</u> comment about his sister's weight just as she was biting into the piece of cake cast a cloud over the birthday celebrations.

Which of the following is the definition for the underlined word in the sentence above?
   a. timely
   b. biting
   c. concerned
   d. effective

---

45. Why is it important to consult more than one source while researching a topic?
   a. It will give you different ideas for wording your argument.
   b. It will help you to validate or dismiss information.
   c. It will show that many different ways exist to look at an issue.
   d. It will prove you have taken your research seriously.

---

46. In *Tom Sawyer,* Tom gets punished for skipping school after he disappoints his aunt. This is how he feels: "Then he betook himself to his seat, rested his elbows on his desk and his jaws in his hands, and stared at the wall with the stony stare of suffering that has reached the limit and can no further go." This means that:
   a. Tom is feeling angry that he was caught skipping school.
   b. Tom is suffering the most pain that any human being could ever feel.
   c. Tom does not understand that what he did was wrong.
   d. Tom feels that his suffering is great, because it is all he thinks about.

The next two questions are based on the following charts.

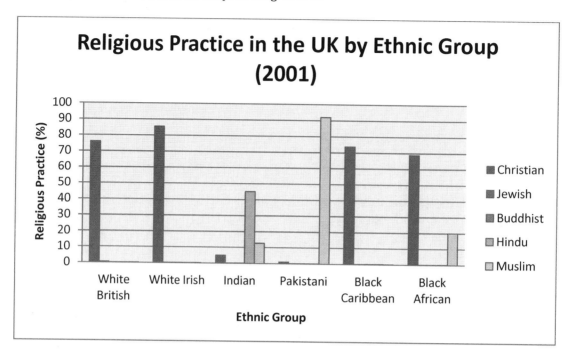

Total Population Numbers by Ethnicity (as of 2001)

White British	White Irish	Indian	Pakistani	Black Caribbean	Black African
50,366,497	691,232	1,053,411	747,285	565,876	485,277

Source: Census 2001

47. As a combined percentage based on population numbers, which religion is most practiced in the United Kingdom?
    a. Christianity
    b. Judaism
    c. Islam
    d. Hinduism

48. According to the charts, which two religions listed on the chart are practiced the least?
    a. Islam and Hinduism
    b. Judaism and Buddhism
    c. Buddhism and Hinduism
    d. Hinduism and Judaism

49. Which of the following statements would be LEAST relevant in a formal essay about artist Salvador Dalí?
   a. Although his works are famed for their dream-like qualities, Dalí executed them with realism reminiscent of the Renaissance masters.
   b. Salvador Dalí's eccentricity extended beyond his artwork, affecting the strange public persona he created, which can be witnessed in his numerous television appearances.
   c. I've always found Dalí's painting The Persistence of Memory to be really disturbing for some reason.
   d. Although Salvador Dalí is best known for his paintings, he also was active in cinema and collaborated with such filmmakers as Luis Bunuel and Alfred Hitchcock.

50. The subject content textbooks that you were given or assigned to use in school are typically examples of which type of information source?
   a. Primary sources
   b. Secondary sources
   c. Tertiary sources only
   d. Any of these equally

The next three questions are based on the following passage:

Black History Month is unnecessary. In a place and time in which we overwhelmingly elected an African American president, we can and should move to a post-racial approach to education. As *Detroit Free Press* columnist Rochelle Riley wrote in a February 1 column calling for an end to Black History Month, "I propose that, for the first time in American history, this country has reached a point where we can stop celebrating separately, stop learning separately, stop being American separately."

In addition to being unnecessary, the idea that African American history should be focused on in a given month suggests that it belongs in that month alone. It is important to instead incorporate African American history into what is taught every day as American history. It needs to be recreated as part of mainstream thought and not as an optional, often irrelevant, side note. We should focus efforts on pushing schools to diversify and broaden their curricula.

There are a number of other reasons to abolish it: first, it has become a shallow commercial ritual that does not even succeed in its (limited and misguided) goal of focusing for one month on a sophisticated, intelligent appraisal of the contributions and experiences of African Americans throughout history. Second, there is a paternalistic flavor to the mandated bestowing of a month in which to study African American history that is overcome if we instead assert the need for a comprehensive curriculum. Third, the idea of Black History Month suggests that the knowledge imparted in that month is for African Americans only, rather than for all people.

51. The author's primary purpose is to:
   a. argue that Black History Month should not be so commercial.
   b. argue that Black History Month should be abolished.
   c. argue that Black History Month should be maintained.
   d. suggest that African American history should be taught in two months rather than just one.

52. It can be inferred that the term "post-racial" in the second sentence is an approach that:
    a. is not based on or organized around concepts of race.
    b. treats race as one factor, but not the most important, in determining an individual's experience.
    c. considers race after considering all other elements of a person's identity.
    d. prohibits discussion of race.

53. Which of the following does the author not give as a reason for abolishing Black History Month?
    a. It has become a shallow ritual.
    b. There is a paternalistic feel to being granted one month of focus.
    c. It suggests that the month's education is only for African Americans.
    d. No one learns anything during the month.

Mathematics

DIRECTIONS: The mathematics practice test you are about to take is multiple-choice with only one correct answer per question. Read each test item and circle your answer on the answer sheet below. When you have completed the practice test, you may check your answers with the answers on the answer key following the test.

Answer Sheet

1.	a	b	c	d		20.	a	b	c	d
2.	a	b	c	d		21.	a	b	c	d
3.	a	b	c	d		22.	a	b	c	d
4.	a	b	c	d		23.	a	b	c	d
5.	a	b	c	d		24.	a	b	c	d
6.	a	b	c	d		25.	a	b	c	d
7.	a	b	c	d		26.	a	b	c	d
8.	a	b	c	d		27.	a	b	c	d
9.	a	b	c	d		28.	a	b	c	d
10.	a	b	c	d		29.	a	b	c	d
11.	a	b	c	d		30.	a	b	c	d
12.	a	b	c	d		31.	a	b	c	d
13.	a	b	c	d		32.	a	b	c	d
14.	a	b	c	d		33.	a	b	c	d
15.	a	b	c	d		34.	a	b	c	d
16.	a	b	c	d		35.	a	b	c	d
17.	a	b	c	d		36.	a	b	c	d
18.	a	b	c	d						
19.	a	b	c	d						

1. If Sara can read 15 pages in 10 minutes, how long will it take her to read 45 pages?
   a. 20 minutes
   b. 30 minutes
   c. 40 minutes
   d. 50 minutes

2. Which fraction is equivalent to 0.375?
   a. $\frac{4}{25}$

   b. $\frac{1}{6}$

   c. $\frac{3}{8}$

   d. $\frac{3}{20}$

3. If Leonard bought 2 packs of batteries for x amount of dollars, how many packs of batteries could he purchase for $5.00 at the same rate?
   a. 10x

   b. $\frac{2}{x}$

   c. 2x

   d. $\frac{10}{x}$

4. Choose the algebraic expression that best represents the following situation: Jeral's test score (J) was 5 points higher than half of Kara's test score (K).
   a. $J = \frac{1}{2}K + 5$

   b. $J = 2K - 5$

   c. $K = \left(J - \frac{1}{2}\right) - 5$

   d. $K = \frac{1}{2}J - 5$

5. Enrique weighs 5 pounds more than twice Brendan's weight. If their total weight is 225 pounds, how much does Enrique weigh?
   a. 125 pounds
   b. 152 pounds
   c. 115 pounds
   d. 165 pounds

6. Which of the following is listed in order from *greatest to least*?

a. $2\frac{1}{4}, \frac{32}{5}, \frac{4}{5}, -5, -2$

b. $\frac{32}{5}, 2\frac{1}{4}, \frac{4}{5}, -2, -5$

c. $-5, -2, \frac{32}{5}, \frac{4}{5}, 2\frac{1}{4}$

d. $\frac{32}{5}, 2\frac{1}{4}, \frac{4}{5}, -5, -2$

---

7. Which of the following is equivalent to $-8 + (17 - 9) \times 4 + 7$?

a. 11

b. 31

c. 28

d. 80

---

8. Olga drew the regular figure shown here. She painted part of the figure a light color and part of it a darker color. She left the rest of the figure white.

Which of the following equations best models the part of the figure Olga left white?

a. $1 - \frac{1}{3} - \frac{1}{3} = \frac{1}{3}$

b. $1 - \frac{1}{6} - \frac{1}{6} = \frac{2}{3}$

c. $1 - \frac{1}{6} - \frac{1}{2} = \frac{1}{3}$

d. $1 - \frac{1}{2} - \frac{1}{3} = \frac{2}{3}$

---

9. The following items were purchased at the grocery store. What was the average price paid for the items?

Item	Cost	Quantity
Milk	$3.50/carton	2
Banana	$0.30 each	5
Can of soup	$1.25/can	3
Carrots	$0.45/stick	6

    a. $0.34
    b. $0.55
    c. $0.93
    d. $1.38

10. A farmer had about 150 bags of potatoes on his trailer. Each bag contained from 23 to 27 pounds of potatoes. Which is the best estimate of the total number of pounds of potatoes on the farmer's trailer?
    a. 3,000
    b. 3,700
    c. 4,100
    d. 5,000

11. A rectangle has a width of 9 inches and a length of 15 inches. If the rectangle is enlarged by a scale factor of $\frac{3}{2}$, what is the perimeter of the dilated rectangle?
    a. 68 inches
    b. 72 inches
    c. 60 inches
    d. 64 inches

12. Find $\left(\frac{27}{9}\right) \times \left(\sqrt{25} \times 2\right)$.
    a. 90
    b. 12
    c. 45
    d. 30

13. Which of the following scenarios can be represented by the equation $14 + x = 52$?
    a. Stella has $14 in her wallet. How much money does she have if she adds the $52 she earned babysitting last night?
    b. Marcus earns $52 mowing yards. How much money does he save if he buys his brother a birthday present that costs $14 and saves the rest?
    c. Troy earns $52 working for a neighbor. How much money does he have if he earns an additional $14 working for his aunt?
    d. Izzy has $14 of money in her piggy bank. How much money does she have if she adds the $52 she receives for her birthday?

14. A building has a number of floors of equal height, as well as a thirty-foot spire above them all. If the height of each floor in feet is h, and there are n floors in the building, which of the following represents the building's total height in feet?
    a. $n + h + 30$
    b. $nh + 30$
    c. $30n + h$
    d. $30h + n$

15. If $x + y > 0$ when $x > y$, which of the following cannot be true?
    a. $x = 3$ and $y = 0$
    b. $x = -3$ and $y = 0$
    c. $x = -4$ and $y = -3$
    d. $x = 3$ and $y = -3$

16. Rick renovated his home. He made his bedroom 40% larger (length and width) than its original size. If the original dimensions were 144 inches by 168 inches, how big is his room now if measured in feet?
    a. 12 ft × 14 ft
    b. 16.8 ft × 19.6 ft
    c. 4.8 ft × 5.6 ft
    d. 201.6 ft × 235.2 ft

17. Which of the following best describes the relationship of this set of data?

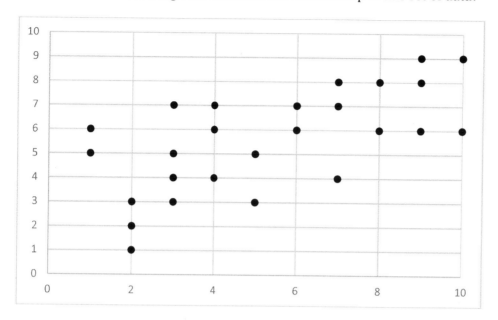

a. High positive correlation
b. Low positive correlation
c. Low negative correlation
d. No correlation

18. A scatterplot is constructed for the data below. Which of the following best describes this data?

Study Time (Minutes)	10	15	20	25
Average Test Scores (%)	60	69	80	89

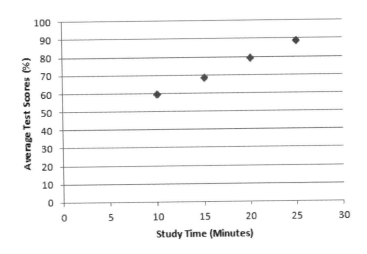

a. This is a linear association with a positive correlation between bivariate data.
b. This is a linear association with a negative correlation between bivariate data.
c. This is a nonlinear association between bivariate data.
d. There is no association between the bivariate data.

19. In the figure below, a circle with radius r is inscribed within a square. What is the area of the shaded region?

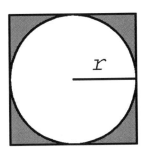

a. $4r - \pi$
b. $(4 - \pi)r^2$
c. $4r^2 - \pi$
d. $4r - \pi r^2$

20. Shaylee goes shopping for two types of fruit: mangoes that cost $2.00 each and coconuts that cost $4.00 each. If she buys 10 pieces of fruit and spends $30.00, how many pieces of each type of fruit did she buy?
    a. 4 mangoes and 6 coconuts
    b. 5 mangoes and 5 coconuts
    c. 6 mangoes and 4 coconuts
    d. 7 mangoes and 3 coconuts

The following question is based on the chart below.

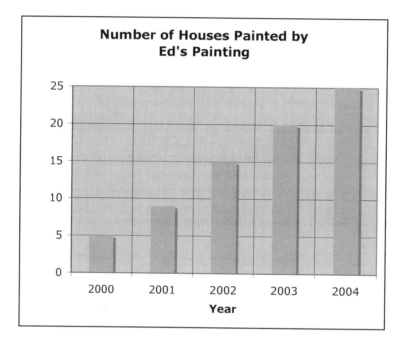

21. What is the approximate average number of houses Ed painted each year from 2000 to 2004?
    a. 15
    b. 74
    c. 12
    d. 22

22. Martin's bed is 7 feet in length. Which of the following represents the length of the bed, in centimeters?
    a. 209.42 cm
    b. 213.36 cm
    c. 215.52 cm
    d. 217.94 cm

23. Curtis measured the temperature of water in a flask in Science class. The temperature of the water was 35°C. He carefully heated the flask so that the temperature of the water increased about 2°C every 3 minutes. Approximately how much had the temperature of the water increased after 20 minutes?

    a. 10°C
    b. 13°C
    c. 15°C
    d. 35°C

The graph below shows Aaron's distance from home at times throughout his morning run. Assume that his route lies along a straight line.

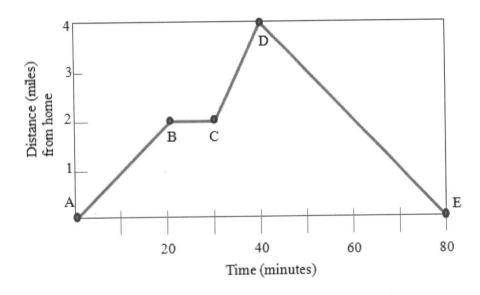

24. Which of the following statements is true?
    a. Aaron ran a total distance of four miles. *no*
    b. Aaron's average speed between points A and D was higher than his average speed between *slower* *no* points D and E.
    c. Aaron rested for ten minutes after running the first thirty minutes. *no*
    d. Aaron's average speed was 6 mph.

25. Trevor is researching the cost of college. The tuition for a two-year (four-semester) program at the community college costs $2,000 per semester. The tuition for a four-year (eight-semester) program at the state college costs $6,000 per semester. Which of the following statements is true regarding the cost of these two programs?
    a. The costs of the two programs are the same.
    b. The four-year program costs twice as much as the two-year program.
    c. The four-year program cost four times as much as the two-year program.
    d. The four-year program costs six times as much as the two-year program.

26. Solve for n in the following equation: $4n - p = 3r$
   a. 3r/4 - p
   b. p + 3r
   c. p - 3r
   d. 3r/4 + p/4

The next three questions are based on the following information:

Mrs. McConnell's Classroom	
Eye Color	**Number of Students**
Brown	14
Blue	9
Hazel	5
Green	2

27. What percentage of students in Mrs. McConnell's classroom have either hazel or green eyes?
   a. 23%
   b. 30%
   c. 47%
   d. 77%

28. How many more students have either brown or blue eyes than students who have hazel or green eyes?
   a. 23
   b. 7
   c. 16
   d. 14

29. What is the ratio of students with brown eyes to students with green eyes?
   a. 1:2
   b. 3:1
   c. 1:5
   d. 7:1

---

30. What is $\dfrac{4\frac{2}{9}}{2\frac{2}{3}}$?

   a. $11\frac{7}{27}$

   b. $1\frac{7}{12}$

   c. $1\frac{1}{12}$

   d. $2\frac{5}{12}$

---

31. On a map, the space of $\frac{1}{2}$ of an inch represents 15 miles. If two cities are $4\frac{3}{5}$ inches apart on the map, what is the actual distance between the two cities?

    a. 138 miles

    b. 39 miles

    c. 23 miles

    d. 125 miles

---

32. If Louis travels on his bike at an average rate of 20 mph, how long will it take him to travel 240 miles?

    a. 48 hours

    b. 12 hours

    c. 20 hours

    d. 8 hours

---

33. Maria paid $28.00 for a jacket that was discounted by 30%. What was the original price of the jacket?

    a. $36.00

    b. $47.60

    c. $40.00

    d. $42.50

---

34. A soda company is testing a new sized can to put on the market. The new can is 6 inches in diameter and 12 inches in height. What is the volume of the can in cubic inches?

    a. 339

    b. 113

    c. 432

    d. 226

---

35. John's Gym charges its members according to the equation $C = 40m$ where m is the number of months and C represents the total cost to each customer after m months. Ralph's Recreation Room charges its members according to the equation $C = 45m$. What relationship can be determined about the monthly cost to the members of each company?

    a. John's monthly membership fee is equal to Ralph's monthly membership fee.

    b. John's monthly membership fee is more than Ralph's monthly membership fee.

    c. John's monthly membership fee is less than Ralph's monthly membership fee.

    d. No relationship between the monthly membership fees can be determined.

36. Which of the following best describes the data represented by this scatterplot?

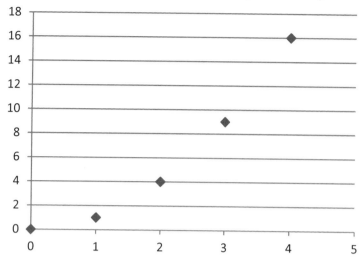

a. This is a linear association with a positive correlation between bivariate data.
b. This is a linear association with a negative correlation between bivariate data.
c. This is a nonlinear association between bivariate data.
d. There is no association between the bivariate data.

Science

DIRECTIONS: The science practice test you are about to take is multiple-choice with only one correct answer per question. Read each test item and circle your answer on the answer sheet below. When you have completed the practice test, you may check your answers with those on the answer key that follows the test.

Answer Sheet

1.	a	b	c	d		28.	a	b	c	d
2.	a	b	c	d		29.	a	b	c	d
3.	a	b	c	d		30.	a	b	c	d
4.	a	b	c	d		31.	a	b	c	d
5.	a	b	c	d		32.	a	b	c	d
6.	a	b	c	d		33.	a	b	c	d
7.	a	b	c	d		34.	a	b	c	d
8.	a	b	c	d		35.	a	b	c	d
9.	a	b	c	d		36.	a	b	c	d
10.	a	b	c	d		37.	a	b	c	d
11.	a	b	c	d		38.	a	b	c	d
12.	a	b	c	d		39.	a	b	c	d
13.	a	b	c	d		40.	a	b	c	d
14.	a	b	c	d		41.	a	b	c	d
15.	a	b	c	d		42.	a	b	c	d
16.	a	b	c	d		43.	a	b	c	d
17.	a	b	c	d		44.	a	b	c	d
18.	a	b	c	d		45.	a	b	c	d
19.	a	b	c	d		46.	a	b	c	d
20.	a	b	c	d		47.	a	b	c	d
21.	a	b	c	d		48.	a	b	c	d
22.	a	b	c	d		49.	a	b	c	d
23.	a	b	c	d		50.	a	b	c	d
24.	a	b	c	d		51.	a	b	c	d
25.	a	b	c	d		52.	a	b	c	d
26.	a	b	c	d		53.	a	b	c	d
27.	a	b	c	d						

1. Which of the following correctly lists the cellular hierarchy from the simplest to the most complex structure?
   a. tissue, cell, organ, organ system, organism
   b. organism, organ system, organ, tissue, cell
   c. organ system, organism, organ, tissue, cell
   d. cell, tissue, organ, organ system, organism

2. What is the first line of defense against invading bacteria?
   a. The skin
   b. Macrophages
   c. T-cells
   d. Lymphocytes

3. What is the longest phase of the cell cycle?
   a. mitosis
   b. cytokinesis
   c. interphase
   d. metaphase

The next two questions are based on the following Punnett square.

B = alleles for brown eyes; g = alleles for green eyes

	B	g
B	BB	Bg
g	Bg	gg

4. Which word describes the allele for green eyes?
   a. dominant
   b. recessive
   c. homozygous
   d. heterozygous

5. What is the possibility that the offspring produced will have brown eyes?
   a. 25%
   b. 50%
   c. 75%
   d. 100%

6. In order to be included in the formation of a scientific conclusion, evidence must be
    a. Quantitative
    b. Reproducible
    c. Obvious
    d. All of the above

7. When does the nuclear division of somatic cells take place during cellular reproduction?
    a. meiosis
    b. cytokinesis
    c. interphase
    d. mitosis

8. Which structure in the brain is responsible for arousal and maintenance of consciousness?
    a. The midbrain
    b. The reticular activating system
    c. The diencephalon
    d. The limbic system

9. The rate of a chemical reaction depends on all of the following except
    a. temperature.
    b. surface area.
    c. presence of catalysts.
    d. amount of mass lost.

10. If an organism is *AaBb*, which of the following combinations in the gametes is impossible?
    a. AB
    b. aa
    c. aB
    d. Ab

11. Scientists often form hypotheses based on particular observations. Which of the following is NOT true of a good hypothesis?
    a. A good hypothesis is complex.
    b. A good hypothesis is testable.
    c. A good hypothesis is logical.
    d. A good hypothesis predicts future events.

12. What is the role of ribosomes?
    a. make proteins
    b. waste removal
    c. transport
    d. storage

13. Which of the following is not provided as a result of the valid research and observations recorded by scientists?
  a. A better understanding of the physical world
  b. The ability to predict possible outcomes affected by actions
  c. The ability to prevent earthquakes and other natural disasters
  d. The creation of various substances and technologies that enhance our world

14. The hydrogen bonds in a water molecule make water a good _____ .
  a. Solvent for lipids
  b. Participant in replacement reactions
  c. Surface for small particles and living organisms to move across
  d. Solvent for polysaccharides such as cellulose

15. Which of the following organ systems has the purpose of producing movement through contraction?
  a. Skeletal
  b. Muscular
  c. Cardiovascular
  d. Respiratory

16. Which of the following statements is *not* true of most metals?
  a. They are good conductors of heat.
  b. They are gases at room temperature.
  c. They are ductile.
  d. They make up the majority of elements on the periodic table.

17. Where does fertilization of an egg by a sperm cell occur?
  a. The ovary
  b. The uterus
  c. The cervix
  d. The fallopian tubes

18. A student's science fair project involves studying the effects of fertilizer on grass height. After four weeks of measuring height weekly, the student was not able to tell any difference between two pots of grass he had fertilized and watered weekly. How could this experiment be improved?
  a. Measure height more frequently
  b. Only water one of the pots
  c. Use a more accurate method of measurement
  d. Only fertilize one of the pots

19. Which of the following is not a type of connective tissue?
    a. smooth
    b. cartilage
    c. adipose tissue
    d. blood tissue

20. Which of the following is considered an intensive property?
    a. mass
    b. weight
    c. volume
    d. density

21. Which of the following correctly describes the trait Ll, if "L" represents tallness and "l" represents shortness?
    a. heterozygous genotype and tall phenotype
    b. heterozygous phenotype and tall genotype
    c. homozygous genotype and short phenotype
    d. homozygous phenotype and short genotype

22. Which of the following statements accurately characterizes the relationship between genes and chromosomes?
    a. Each gene contains multiple chromosomes.
    b. Each chromosome contains multiple genes.
    c. Genes and chromosomes are two words for the same thing.
    d. Genes and chromosomes are not the same thing, but always occur in equal numbers.

23. Which of the following is a constant?
    a. The freezing point of water
    b. The temperature at which iron ore will melt
    c. The human population size
    d. The time the sun rises each day

24. Which organ system includes the spleen?
    a. Endocrine
    b. Lymphatic
    c. Respiratory
    d. Digestive

25. Which of the following statements describes the function of smooth muscle tissue?
    a. It contracts to force air into and out of the lungs.
    b. It contracts to force air into and out of the stomach.
    c. It contracts to support the spinal column.
    d. It contracts to assist the stomach in the mechanical breakdown of food.

26. Which part of the cardiac conduction system is the most distal from the initial impulse generation and actually conducts the charge throughout the heart tissue?
    a. SA node
    b. AV node
    c. Perkinje fibers
    d. Bundle of His

27. Which cells are found in the skin and assist in boosting immune function?
    a. Melanocytes
    b. Reticular fibers
    c. Eccrine glands
    d. Langerhans cells

28. Which of the following compose the central nervous system?
    a. the brain and spinal cord
    b. the brain and heart
    c. the heart and lungs
    d. all the muscles in the body

29. Afferent lymph vessels carry lymph:
    a. toward the spleen
    b. away from the spleen
    c. toward the lymph node
    d. away from the lymph node

30. Which of the following is usually the first form of study in a new area of scientific inquiry?
    a. descriptive studies
    b. controlled experiments
    c. choosing a method and design
    d. identifying dependent and independent variables

31. The primary function of which biological system is to move nutrients and chemicals through the body?
    a. Circulatory
    b. Digestive
    c. Respiratory
    d. Urinary

---

32. What is the proper order of the divisions of the small intestine as food passes through the gastrointestinal tract?
    a. Ileum, duodenum, jejunum
    b. Duodenum, Ileum, jejunum
    c. Duodenum, jejunum, ileum
    d. Ileum, jejunum, duodenum

---

33. Two isotopes of the same molecule have different numbers of _____.
    a. Electrons
    b. Protons
    c. Neutrons
    d. Nuclei

---

34. The diaphragm belongs in which of the following biological systems?
    a. Circulatory
    b. Nervous
    c. Respiratory
    d. Skeletal

---

35. What function do platelets serve in the bloodstream?
    a. They carry nutrients from food.
    b. They carry oxygen.
    c. They form blood clots to stop bleeding.
    d. They destroy pathogens and other foreign materials.

---

36. What is the term for the gap between neurons, where hormones and other messenger ions can pass from one cell to the next?
    a. Axon
    b. Dendrite
    c. Ganglion
    d. Synapse

37. Which of the following is NOT one of the three types of muscle found in the human body?
    a. Cardiac
    b. Nodular
    c. Skeletal
    d. Smooth

38. Which of the following terms is used to describe muscular contractions that move food material through the digestive tract?
    a. Homeostasis
    b. Ingestion
    c. Metastasis
    d. Peristalsis

39. What laboratory practice can increase the accuracy of a measurement?
    a. repeating the measurement several times
    b. calibrating the equipment each time you use it
    c. using metric measuring devices
    d. reading the laboratory instructions before the lab

40. What is the term for the region of the body that lies below the ribcage and above the pelvis?
    a. Abdomen
    b. Peritoneum
    c. Thorax
    d. Umbilicus

41. Which of the following is true of skeletal muscle tissue?
    a. Skeletal muscle tissue consists of elongated, spindle-shaped cells, each of which contains a single nucleus.
    b. Skeletal muscle tissue consists of cross-striated, quadrangular cells, each of which contains a single nucleus.
    c. Skeletal muscle tissue consists of striated, cylindrical fibers, each of which contains nuclei located towards the outer edges of the fiber.
    d. Skeletal muscle tissue consists of tightly packed, cuboidal cells, each of which contains a single nucleus.

42. What disorder results from a hypersensitivity of the immune system?
    a. Allergy
    b. Asthma
    c. Cancer
    d. Fever

43. Which of the following is NOT a function of the nervous system?
    a. Processing and integrating sensory input
    b. Extracting information about the environment
    c. Sending signals to the muscles to induce contraction
    d. Regulating the body through hormonal production

44. During which part of the menstrual cycle is a woman MOST likely to become pregnant?
    a. During menstruation
    b. At ovulation
    c. Halfway between the end of menstruation and the onset of ovulation
    d. A woman is equally fertile at any point in her menstrual cycle

45. What is the name for a joint that can only move in two directions?
    a. hinge
    b. insertion
    c. ball and socket
    d. flange

46. Which force motivates filtration in the kidneys?
    a. osmosis
    b. smooth muscle contraction
    c. peristalsis
    d. blood pressure

47. What is the function of the Golgi apparatus?
    a. It contains the cell's genetic material.
    b. It helps maintain the cell's shape and structural integrity.
    c. It prepares proteins and other large molecules for transport to other parts of the cell.
    d. It is responsible for cellular metabolism, producing the energy used by other organelles.

48. Which hormone is *not* secreted by a gland in the brain?
    a. Human chorionic gonadotropin (HCG)
    b. Gonadotropin releasing hormone (GnRH)
    c. Luteinizing hormone (LH)
    d. Follicle stimulating hormone (FSH)

49. What is the term for the process by which unspecialized cells transform into more specialized cells?
    a. Differentiation
    b. Evolution
    c. Mitosis
    d. Synthesis

50. Where are the vocal cords located?
    a. bronchi
    b. trachea
    c. larynx
    d. epiglottis

A biology student is studying the effects of acid rain on tomato plants. He plants four tomato plants in identical pots, using the same type of soil to fill each pot. He places the pots together in the same location. They receive the same amount of sunlight and water each day. The only difference is the pH of the water used to water the plants. The first plant receives water with a neutral pH of 7, which will allow the student to better determine the effects of giving plants water that is more acidic. The second plant receives water with a pH of 5. The third receives water with a pH of 3. The fourth receives water with a pH of 1.

51. Which of the following is a serious flaw in the design of this experiment?
    a. The experiment has only one variable.
    b. The experiment has several constants.
    c. The experiment has no repetition.
    d. The experiment has no control.

Two balances in a classroom laboratory are used to determine the mass of an object. The actual mass of the object is 15.374 grams.

Measurement	Triple Beam Balance	Digital Balance
1	15.38 grams	15.375 grams
2	15.39 grams	15.376 grams
3	15.37 grams	15.376 grams
4	15.38 grams	15.375 grams

52. Which of the following statements is true concerning the accuracy and precision of these two balances?
    a. The triple beam balance is both more accurate and more precise.
    b. The triple beam balance is more accurate, but the digital balance is more precise.
    c. The digital balance is more accurate, but the triple beam balance is more precise.
    d. The digital balance is both more accurate and more precise.

---

53. In mammals, blood pH must be kept fairly constant (very close to 7.4) in order for these animals to survive. Which two organs play the MOST IMPORTANT role in regulating blood pH in mammals?
    a. kidneys and lungs
    b. heart and lungs
    c. kidneys and liver
    d. liver and lungs

English and Language Usage

DIRECTIONS: The English and language usage practice test you are about to take is multiple-choice with only one correct answer per question. Read each test item and circle your answer on the answer sheet below. When you have completed the practice test, you may check your answers with those answers on the answer key that follows the test.

Answer Sheet

1.	a	b	c	d		15.	a	b	c	d
2.	a	b	c	d		16.	a	b	c	d
3.	a	b	c	d		17.	a	b	c	d
4.	a	b	c	d		18.	a	b	c	d
5.	a	b	c	d		19.	a	b	c	d
6.	a	b	c	d		20.	a	b	c	d
7.	a	b	c	d		21.	a	b	c	d
8.	a	b	c	d		22.	a	b	c	d
9.	a	b	c	d		23.	a	b	c	d
10.	a	b	c	d		24.	a	b	c	d
11.	a	b	c	d		25.	a	b	c	d
12.	a	b	c	d		26.	a	b	c	d
13.	a	b	c	d		27.	a	b	c	d
14.	a	b	c	d		28.	a	b	c	d

1. Writing, doing yoga, and _____ were her favorite activities.
    a. playing volleyball
    b. doing volleyball
    c. making volleyball
    d. volleyballing

2. Which sentence is written correctly?
    a. The student, who was caught cheating, was given detention.
    b. The student who was caught cheating was given detention.
    c. The student who was caught cheating, was given detention.
    d. The student; who was caught cheating; was given detention.

3. Which sentence is written most clearly?
    a. His neighbor's dog was walked for an allowance by the boy.
    b. The boy walked his neighbor's dog for an allowance.
    c. For an allowance, the boy walked the dog of his neighbor's.
    d. The dog of his neighbor's was walked by the boy for an allowance.

4. Every kid in the neighborhood has _____ own bicycle.
    a. its
    b. their
    c. our
    d. her

5. In composing an essay or similar piece, in which sequence should a writer do the following?
    a. List all details supporting each main point, organize details in sequential order, narrow topics to a main idea, find which main points support the main idea, decide how to sequence main points
    b. Decide how to sequence main points, narrow topics to a main idea, find which main points support the main idea, organize details in sequential order, list all details supporting each main point
    c. Organize details in sequential order, decide how to sequence main points, list all details supporting each main point, narrow topics to a main idea, find which main points support the main idea
    d. Narrow topics to a main idea, find which main points support the main idea, decide how to sequence main points, list all details supporting each main point, organize details in sequential order

"Because he was late, he missed the field trip, and this caused him to fail the class."

6. In this sentence which numbers and kinds of clauses are included?
    a. One dependent clause and one independent clause
    b. Two dependent clauses and one independent clause
    c. One dependent clause and two independent clauses
    d. Two dependent clauses and two independent clauses

7. Of the following versions of this sentence, which one has a complex structure?
    a. You will have to come back tomorrow; you arrived later than the deadline today.
    b. You will have to come back tomorrow since you arrived past the deadline today.
    c. You arrived following the deadline today and will have to come back tomorrow.
    d. You arrived late, which was after the deadline; you must come back tomorrow.

8. Based on vocabulary words you can think of beginning with *trans-*, what does this prefix mean?
    a. Across
    b. Change
    c. Carrying
    d. Different

The impoverished shepherds stumbled upon the stele while desperately searching for some lost sheep; they were surprised and puzzled by the bizarre lines and squiggles that covered its face.

9. Which of the following choices best defines the underlined word?
    a. an item that has been looted from a tomb
    b. a sign that indicates direction
    c. the side of cliff
    d. a large, inscribed stone

10. Which of the following choices is NOT an appropriate way to express an opinion in a formal debate?
    a. There are still a variety of arguments concerning the nature of space-time, and whether Einstein's theory of relativity is applicable in every natural situation.
    b. The study of climate science is an ever-evolving area, but it is important to recognize that the tools being utilized have been tested in other fields.
    c. Energy independence is an important topic that needs to be addressed in a thoughtful, careful manner.
    d. It is the height of hypocrisy to acknowledge that global warming is a problem and then still tool around in a gas-guzzling car.

I often have heard arguments claiming that complete freedom of speech could lead to dangerous situations. Without complete freedom of speech, we hardly are living in a free society.

11. Which word would best link these sentences?
    a. However
    b. Therefore
    c. So
    d. Supposedly

---

12. After the lecture had officially ended, the professor surprised his students by <u>defaming</u> the guest speakers he had invited. Which of the following substitutions creates a more negative connotation of the underlined word?
    a. gently mocking
    b. mixing up
    c. embarrassing
    d. vilifying

---

13. Which of the following is essential in a concluding statement of an argument?
    a. The introduction of new points that might lead to future arguments.
    b. A summary of the issue that reinforces clearly its main points.
    c. A contradiction of the argument's main points to provide fresh perspectives.
    d. An unrelated detail that might lighten the audience's mood after a heated debate.

---

14. Which of the following sentences uses correct punctuation?
    a. The forest was dark and green, it also smelled like pine.
    b. I walked through the carnival quickly, and cautiously.
    c. Jase was older than Mark, but he was not older than Joe.
    d. The horse knows how the path follows the river; and can guide you to the camp.

Amy happily accepted the bouquet of flowers.

15. What does the adverb in the sentence refer to?
    a. how Amy accepted the flowers
    b. where Amy was when she accepted the flowers
    c. the type of flowers Amy accepted
    d. what happened after Amy accepted the flowers

After being kidnapped and held for 10 days, Margaret entreated her captors to release her.

16. The word "entreated" in the sentence above most nearly means what?

    a. threw
    b. sympathized
    c. pleaded
    d. angered

---

17. If the word "antibacterial" describes a substance that kills bacteria, you can infer that the prefix "anti" means
    a. original to
    b. against
    c. before
    d. under

Preparing for the vocabulary test was a test of patience and a lot of hard work, but all my studying paid off in the end with my high score.

18. Which is the most effective way to rewrite the sentence?

    a. All of my studying paid off, even though studying for my vocabulary test was a test of my patience and a lot of hard work.
    b. In the end, preparing for the vocabulary test was a test of patience and took a lot of hard work, but all my studying paid off in my score.
    c. It took a lot of hard work and patience to study for my vocabulary test, but my high score made it all worth it in the end.
    d. My high score on my vocabulary test proved that all of my studying and hard work were a test for me, but one that paid off.

---

19. Which of the following words is spelled correctly?
    a. abbreviate
    b. interum
    c. imbellish
    d. fulcurm

Being the type of guy to hold a grudge after a bad breakup, there was no doubt that Max would refuse the invitation to his ex-girlfriend's wedding.

20. Which answer choice is the best correction for the following sentence?
    a. The invitation to his ex-girlfriend's wedding caused Max to remember that he was the type of guy who holds a grudge.
    b. Max refused the invitation to his ex-girlfriend's wedding.
    c. Being the type of guy to hold a grudge after a bad breakup, I didn't doubt that Max would refuse the invitation to his ex-girlfriend's wedding.
    d. Being the type of guy to hold a grudge after a bad breakup, Max refused the invitation to his ex-girlfriend's wedding.

Aware that his decision would affect the rest of his life, the college Ben chose was Harvard.

21. What is the grammatical error in the sentence?
    a. The subject and the verb do not agree.
    b. The sentence ends with a preposition.
    c. There is a dangling modifier.
    d. There is no error.

---

22. Which of the following is an example of a compound sentence?
    a. I sat outside the room.
    b. Anton needed to get to school, but he first had to stop at the store and pick up some napkins.
    c. Laura reminded her husband that the rent was due, and she looked up their checking account balance online.
    d. Because there was no time to plan for a party, we decided to cancel my birthday celebrations.

---

23. Which sentence is punctuated correctly?
    a. We were uncertain about the terrain ahead; and had lost the map.
    b. These were the items on the shopping list: eggs, milk, bread, peanut butter, and jelly.
    c. Is there any way that we can meet later.
    d. Mary had an appointment at 3 p.m.; George had one at 4 p.m.

It is an unfortunate axiom of nationhood that <u>adjacent</u> states are the most likely to serve as foes rather than allies due to competition over natural resources.

24. Which of the following substitutions best captures the meaning of the underlined word?
    a. sharing a language
    b. sharing ethnicity
    c. touching
    d. distant

25. The words "extraterrestrial" and "terrain" both have the root word "terra" in common. What does "terra" mean?
    a. Sky
    b. Earth
    c. Outside
    d. Inside

My neighbor's pit bull puppy is <u>protective</u>.

26. In this statement, the underlined word is:
    a. A predicate adjective
    b. A predicate nominative
    c. A predictive phrase
    d. The object of a preposition

---

27. Which of the following choices is misspelled?
    a. conciliatory
    b. paroxism
    c. malevolence
    d. pernicious

The teacher often tried to get his quieter students to <u>elaborate on</u> their ideas by asking them concrete questions which served to flush out minutiae and descriptions.

28. Which of the following substitutions best captures the meaning of the underlined words?
    a. improve
    b. add details to
    c. question
    d. examine again

Answers and Explanations #1

Reading Test

1. D: In the third sentence of this passage, the author mentions that wood fences, hedges, and stone walls were in use before the introduction of barbed wire.

2. D: In the first sentence of this passage, the author notes that the introduction of barbed wire came in the late 1800s. The 1800s can also be labeled as the 19th century.

3. D: The survey has the greatest number of participants, so it will be the most accurate in reporting what fruit children like best.

4. B: **Boldface** is a text feature most often used to indicate words that are also listed and defined in the glossary, emphasizing them so students notice them more easily and know they can look up their definitions. A footnote (a) is indicated by a superscript number[1] at the end of the word or sentence, not by **boldface.** Captions (c) below or beside visuals, explaining them, are not in **boldface.** Neither is the text in sidebars (d), i.e., boxes at one side of a page with added information, often in more focus or depth.

5. B: An "onslaught" (a) literally means a vigorous attack or onset, as of criticism here. A "throng" (c) literally means a multitude of people or things assembled/crowded together, as of onlookers here. "Belligerent" literally means hostile, and "mob" (d) literally means an unruly crowd. However, "avalanche" (b) literally means a large snow or ice slide; figuratively it means any sudden, overwhelming amount or occurrence, as with rumors here.

6. D. The passage indicates that the formula increases or boosts the absorption of minerals in the body.

7. B. The directions say to mix equal parts of all the herbs listed.

8. D. The dosage indicates not to exceed four tablespoons in a 24-hour period, so the patient should take it no more than every six hours.

9. C: Persuasive. The author is hoping to persuade or convince young readers to avoid sex by providing them with facts as well as by using rhetorical devices such as dispelling opposing arguments.

10. D: Even printed sources can contain mistakes or outdated information. The best way to evaluate the accuracy of the information in a particular source is to check it against discussions of the same topic in other sources. The information that appears in the most sources likely will be the most accurate.

11. C: "Light as a feather" is a simile, an explicit comparison using "like" or "as." The others are all metaphors, implicit comparisons without "like" or "as," simply referring to something as something else. These are all figures of speech because the meanings are not literal: the stomach has a fluttery feeling, not actual butterflies (a); one does not climb an actual ladder to success (b); the lightweight thing or person does not match a feather's weight (c); meeting a sales quota does not involve physically shooting or hitting a target (d).

12. D: The point of the article is that to maintain good health, a flu vaccine is required annually. Choice 1 can be eliminated. Although the article mentions people older than 50 as needing a vaccine, that group is not the only one. Choice 2 is also incorrect. There is no indication of the need for free vaccines in the piece. Option 3 is not correct. The article states that flu activity peaks in January, making September only the first available date for a flu vaccine.

13. A: A primary characteristic of informative or explanatory writing is that the author assumes certain things to be factual or true. From these assumptions, the author proceeds to inform readers, explain things to them, and offer them insights. Descriptive (b) writing uses multiple sensory details to paint a picture for readers so they can feel they are experiencing what is described. Persuasive (c) writing endeavors to convince readers something is true rather than assuming it is. Narrative (d) writing relates a story or stories to readers.

14. C: The time required for ecological succession to occur indicates that it is a gradual process, not a rapid one. This eliminates choices A and B. The fact that the diagram shows different plants reentering the ecosystem at different times indicates that succession is an orderly process, not a random one. This eliminates choice D. Therefore, the correct choice is C.

15. C: The author states in paragraph 3, "reality television does not display the state of which life actually exists." Throughout the essay, the narrator discusses the ways in which reality television does not reflect reality.

16. A: In this statement, the author is providing a factual definition of a word.

17. B: In paragraph 4, the author explains her assumptions that viewers relate more to real people than actors. "It is as if the viewer can relate more to the show that he or she is watching, because it is real people put in fake situations rather than fake people and characters acting in life-like situations."

18. D: Global environmental protection relates to measures that expand beyond a single neighborhood, forest, or area that might have been damaged by illegal garbage dumping. Scientifically supported statistics about environmental damage throughout the world addresses the global impact of pollution and is not as subjective as a personal story or editorial.

19. B: The advertisement states that Power Fruit contains 100% of the daily value of vitamin C, which means that it meets the amount of vitamin C a person needs each day. The ad also states that Power Fruit contains 35 mg of caffeine, but there is no indication of what the daily value of caffeine is. There is no mention of vitamin A or iron anywhere in the advertisement.

20. D: Lisa and Regina are the only pair whose ads *both* advised that they would be available for weekend childcare.

21. D: No one but Regina fits the family's needs. Lisa will only watch 3 kids, James wants full-time work, and Jose is only available for occasional babysitting.

22. C: James' ad notes that he would consider cooking in addition to childcare.

23. B: We can infer Jose is the youngest from the information in his ad that he is a high-school junior.

24. D: "Crash" and "bribe" have negative connotations, as they are associated with actions that cause destruction or are criminal. "Employ" has a neutral connotation, since it means to use or to give one a job. "Chic" has a positive connotation, as it is used to describe someone or something that is fashionable or desired by others.

25. D: The passage does mention that Helen graduated from Radcliffe College (choice A), and the passage does tell about Anne's role as Helen's teacher (choice B), but the passage as a whole does not focus on Helen's time at college or Anne's life outside of her role as teacher. The passage does not mention services available for the deaf and blind (choice C). The passage does tell about Helen Keller's life.

26. C: The author's use of the phrase "Helen learned at an incredible rate" and the word "remarkable" to describe Helen's life are two examples of the author's admiration.

27. A: A letter in the science journal *Climatic Change* that includes results from some research on fracking showing that it may be more damaging to the environment than burning coal. Only this choice uses science-based research to back up an argument. All of the other choices involve emotional or inconclusive approaches to the issue.

28. C: *An Overview of Persian Society*: a book written by a historian
While the other sources may have reliable information, a book on the research topic is usually a good way to start. Books typically get researched by the author and then vetted by a team of editors. A printed book is more likely to contain accurate information than a webpage. A blog can contain accurate information, but the blog listed in Choice B is not written by an expert in the field. Choice D is too narrow for the topic at hand.

29. D: While it is true that most students do not go to college, and that working is beneficial, attending school until 18 is valuable. At 16, most students do not really know what they want to do: if they drop out of school early, they may regret that they lost the chance to study hard and attend college. Research shows that college grads make more money than those with less education.

This choice provides a counterclaim while acknowledging the truth in the speaker's argument. Choice A opens with an ad hominem attack and fails to assert a counterclaim. Choice B lacks a counterclaim. Choice C lacks an acknowledgment of what the speaker claimed.

30. B: The California Update notes state that the upcoming election will be discussed.

31. C: Smart Talk lists a discussion about President Obama's first 100 days in office.

32. B: The environment will most likely be discussed most in a program on green jobs.

33. D: This statement is most likely to be made in a show on graffiti.

34. C: People in government knew that the purchase would make the country more powerful, but the last sentence specifically states that they needed to explore. Answer choice C is the best prediction of what would occur next. Answer choices A and D infer too much, since you cannot assume any of these based on this passage given. Answer choice B is simply a statement that does not predict anything for the future.

35. A: While all of the answer choices are in the passage, only answer choice A answers the question as it is written. The desire to become more powerful is listed in the passage as one of the reasons that the United States decided to buy the land.

36. D: The reader can use the word "excited" to help infer that the best synonym for "astounded" is "shocked".

37. C: The Eagle Eye Trail is the only trail that does not connect to one of the other trails.

38. A. The Beaverton Falls trail is an easy trail and says that it is suitable for people of all ages. It also offers picnic areas. The other trails listed are moderate to hard and do not offer areas to picnic.

39. D. According to the table, the Toulanne Trail offers boat rentals as early as May; whereas, the Silver Bullet Trail does not allow fishing until July.

40. C. The total distance they will hike is 2.6 miles + 9.5 miles = 12.1 miles. If they hike 3 miles per hour, it will take them $\frac{12.1}{3}$ = 4.03 hours to hike 12.1 miles.

41. B. The seven steps of instructions result in the word *amoral*.

42. C. Among the answer choices, only the word *deject* would appear between the words *degressive* and *delectation*. The words *deligacy* (answer choice A) and *delirium* (answer choice D) would follow the word *delectation*. The word *degrade* (answer choice B) would precede the word *degressive*.

43. D: The purpose of narrative (a) writing is storytelling. Even when authors want to afford insights and/or teach lessons as well as entertain readers, they accomplish their purposes through storytelling. The purposes of expository (b) writing are to inform, explain, and/or direct readers. The purpose of persuasive (c) writing is to convince readers to believe or agree with the author's position and/or argument. The purpose of speculative (d) writing is to encourage readers to explore ideas and potential responses rather than entertain, tell stories, inform, explain, direct, or convince.

44. B. The context of the sentence indicates that Calvin's comment is anything but kind, so the closest adjective in this case is *biting*. There is nothing *timely* about his comment, at least in the sense of it being appropriate, so answer choice A is incorrect. The context does not indicate that Calvin is *concerned* so much as critical, so answer choice C is incorrect. And the sentence in no way indicates that Calvin's remark is *effective*, so answer choice D is incorrect.

45. B: Even printed sources can be wrong sometimes. By cross-referencing your research and consulting more than one source, you can find out whether a source is reliable. Such effort is particularly important when conducting Internet research, since a good deal of information on the Internet is incorrect. Although consulting more than one source may give you different ideas of how to word your argument or show that many different ways to look at an issue, these reasons are not quite as important as validating and dismissing information.

46. D: Tom is caught up in his own guilt, so he thinks that he is suffering more than he actually is.

47. A. The chart indicates that, as a combined percentage based on population numbers, Christianity was most practiced in the United Kingdom. While there are four ethnic groups that practice Christianity as a primary religion (white British, white Irish, black Caribbean, and black African), the population of three of these ethnic groups is fairly small. It is the white British population, and the fact that more than 70% of this population practices Christianity, that made Christianity the primary religion in the United Kingdom.

48. B. Judaism and Buddhism represent the lowest percentage of practice in the United Kingdom, so answer choice B is correct. Among the various ethnic groups, the percent of practitioners in each of these religions is less than 1 percent. Answer choice A is incorrect, because Islam and Hinduism could be considered the second and third most practiced religions on the United Kingdom. The presence of Hinduism in answer choices C and D means that both of these answer choices cannot be correct.

49. C: Use of the first-person point of view and a reliance on personal opinion creates an informal tone. A formal essay should be written in the third-person and rely on assertions supported by research rather than upon vague personal opinions.

50. B: Subject content textbooks in math, social studies, history, sciences, English language arts, etc. are typically secondary sources. Primary sources (a) are used in school too; but they are original works, e.g. novels, books of poetry, books of short stories, plays, etc. for English language arts; or firsthand accounts like journals, diaries, letters, news reports or articles, etc. written during the time period studied for history, which you may have been assigned to read in school along with subject textbooks. You probably also used tertiary sources (c) in school, but as references—e.g. encyclopedias, bibliographies, abstracts, etc.

51. B: The entire passage makes the argument that Black History Month should be abolished, offering various reasons why this is the best course of action.

52. A: The context of the sentence suggests that post-racial refers to an approach in which race is not a useful or positive organizing principle.

53. D: The author of Passage 1 never suggests that people do not learn about African American history during Black History Month.

Mathematics Test

1.B. The relationship can be expressed as: $\frac{15}{10} = \frac{45}{x}$; $15x = 450$; $x = 30$.

2. C: Changing 0.375 into a fraction by writing $\frac{375}{1000}$ because 0.375 is in the thousandths. Then reduce the fraction by dividing the numerator and the denominator by the greatest common factor of 125 to get $\frac{3}{8}$.

3. D. First set the relationship up and solve for the number of packs: $\frac{x}{2} = \frac{5}{packs}$; $x(packs) = 10$; packs $= \frac{10}{x}$.

4. A. The correct expression is: $J = \frac{1}{2}K + 5$.

5. B. If E + B = 225, and E = 2B + 5, then 225 – B = 2B + 5. Solving for B, 3B = 220 and B = 73.3. 225 – 73.3 = 151.7.

6. B: The rational numbers for Choice B can be compared by either converting all of them to decimals or finding common denominators and comparing the newly written fractions. Using the first approach, the rational numbers shown for Choice B in order from left to right can be written as 6.4, 2.25, and 0.80. These numbers are indeed written in order from greatest to least. Also, the integer –2 is greater than –5. Thus, the numbers, $\frac{32}{5}, 2\frac{1}{4}, \frac{4}{5}, -2, -5$, are listed in order from greatest to least.

7. B: The order of operations requires evaluation of the expression inside the parentheses as a first step. Thus, the expression can be re-written as $-8 + 8 \times 4 + 7$. Now, the order of operations next requires all multiplications and divisions to be computed as they appear from left to right. Thus, the expression can be written as $-8 + 32 + 7$. Finally, the addition may be computed as it appears from left to right. The expression simplifies to $24 + 7$, or 31.

8. C: To answer this question, notice that this figure is a regular hexagon, having 6 equal sides and angles. The part painted darker can be represented by $\frac{1}{6}$. The part painted lighter is clearly $\frac{1}{2}$, which is equivalent to $\frac{3}{6}$. The whole figure is represented by the number 1. So, 1 minus $\frac{1}{6}$ minus $\frac{3}{6}$ equals $\frac{2}{6}$ which is equivalent to $\frac{1}{3}$. Therefore, the equation, $1 - \frac{1}{6} - \frac{1}{2} = \frac{1}{3}$ best models the part of the figure Olga left white.

9. C. Calculate the average price as $\frac{((3.5 \times 2) + (0.3 \times 5) + (1.25 \times 3) + (0.45 \times 6))}{(2 + 5 + 3 + 6)} = 0.93$.

10. B: 3,700 is the only answer between the minimum number of potatoes that could have been on the trailer, 150 × 23 = 3,450, and the maximum number of potatoes that could have been on the trailer, 27 × 150 = 4,050. Another method that could be used to answer this question is to multiply 25, the number halfway between 23 and 27, by 150. The product, 3,750 is very near the correct answer.

11. B: The width of the enlarged rectangle is equal to the product of 9 in and $\frac{3}{2}$, or 13.5 in. The length of the enlarged rectangle is equal to the product of 15 in and $\frac{3}{2}$, or 22.5 in. $Perimeter_{rectangle} = 2w + 2l$. Thus, the perimeter is equal to 2×13.5 in + 2×22.5 in = 72 in.

12. D. Remember the order of operations: $\left(\frac{27}{9}\right) = 3$ and $\left(\sqrt{25} \times 2\right) = 10$; 3 × 10 = 30.

13. B: Let x represent the amount of money saved, $52 the amount earned mowing yards, and $14 the amount spent on a birthday present. Then $52 – $14 = x. This can be rearranged as $14 + x = 52$. Therefore, choice B is correct.

14. B: If there are n floors, and each floor has a height of h feet, then to find the total height of the floors, we just multiply the number of floors by the height of each floor: nh. To find the total height of the building, we must also add the height of the spire, 30 feet. So, the building's total height in feet is $nh + 30$.

15. D: First, test each expression to see which satisfies the condition $x > y$. This condition is met for all the answer choices except B and C, so these need not be considered further. Next, test the remaining choices to see which satisfy the inequality $x + y > 0$. It can be seen that this inequality holds for choice A, but not for choice D, since $x + y = 3 + (-3) = 3 - 3 = 0$ In this case the sum $x + y$ is not greater than 0.

16. B. 144×0.40 = 57.6 + 144 = 201.6 and 168×0.40 = 67.2 + 168 = 235.2; then, convert to feet: $\frac{201.6}{12} = 16.8$ ft and $\frac{235.2}{12} = 19.6$ ft.

17. B: Since the points in this scatterplot "tend" to be rising, this is a positive correlation. However, since the points are not clustered to resemble a straight line, this is a low positive correlation.

18. A: The data form a line that slopes up to the right. Since the data forms a line, there is a linear association between study time and average test score. Since the line slopes up to the right, the linear association has a positive correlation. Therefore, choice A is correct.

19. B: Since the square is circumscribed, its side is twice the length of the radius, or $2r$, and its area is $4r^2$. The area of the circle is given by πr^2. The shaded area is the difference between these two, or $4r^2 - \pi r^2 = (4 - \pi)r^2$.

20. B. If mangoes are represented by x and coconuts are represented by y, then:
x + y = 10, and 2x + 4y = 30
2(10-y) + 4y = 30
20 – 2y + 4y = 30
2y = 10
y = 5 and x = 5, or 5 of each type of fruit

21. A. The average number of houses painted is: $\frac{5 + 9 + 15 + 20 + 25}{5} = 14.8 \approx 15$.

22. B: Since 7 feet equals 84 inches, and 1 inch equals 2.54 centimeters, the following proportion can be written: $\frac{84}{x} = \frac{1}{2.54}$. Solving for x gives: $x = 213.36$. Thus, the bed is 213.36 centimeters in length.

23. B: The water temperature increased by about 2° every 3 minutes, or $\frac{2}{3}$ of a degree every minute. Multiplying the increase in degrees per minute by the total number of minutes yields

$$\frac{2°}{3 \text{ min}} \times 20 \text{ min} = \frac{40}{3}, \text{ or } 13.33°$$

Since the problem asks for the increase in temperature and not the total temperature that results after the increases, 13 is the closest to our answer.

24. D: Notice that the y-axis does not show total distance traveled but rather Aaron's displacement from home. Aaron ran four miles out from home and then back home again, so he ran a total of eight miles. Completing the run in 80 minutes gives him an average speed of:

$$\frac{8 \text{ miles}}{80 \text{ minutes} \times \frac{1 \text{ hour}}{60 \text{ minutes}}} = 6 \text{ mph}$$

25. D: The total cost of the two-year program at the community college is 4($2000), or $8000. The total cost of the four-year program at the state college is 8($6000), or $48,000. Since (6)($8,000) equals $48,000, the cost of the four-year program is six times the cost of the two-year program. Therefore, choice D is correct.

26. D: To solve for n, you have to isolate that variable by putting all of the other terms of the equation, including coefficients, integers, and variables on the other side of the equal sign. Add p to each side of the equation:

$4n - p = 3r$
$4n - p\ (+\ p) = 3r\ (+\ p)$
$4n = 3r + p$

Divide each term by 4:
$\frac{4n}{4} = \frac{3r}{4} + \frac{p}{4}$
$n = \frac{3r}{4} + \frac{p}{4}$

27. A. Total number of students = 14 + 9 + 5 + 2 = 30. Total number of students with either green or hazel eyes: 5 + 2 = 7. To convert the fraction into a percentage: $\frac{7}{30} = \frac{x}{100}$. 700 = 30x. x = 23.3.

28. C. 14 brown + 9 blue = 23; 5 hazel + 2 green = 7; 23 (blue+brown)– 7 (hazel+green) = 16 more blue- or brown-eyed students than hazel- or green-eyed students.

29. D. Brown eyes = 14 and Green eyes = 2. So, the ratio of blue-eyed students to green-eyed students is 14:2 or 7:1.

30. B. $4\frac{2}{9} = \frac{38}{9}$ and $2\frac{2}{3} = \frac{8}{3}$; $\frac{38}{9} \div \frac{8}{3} = \frac{38}{9} \times \frac{3}{8} = \frac{114}{72} = \frac{57}{36} = \frac{19}{12} = 1\frac{7}{12}$.

31. A. $\frac{\frac{1}{2}}{15} = \frac{4\frac{3}{5}}{x}$; $\frac{1}{2}x = 15 \times \frac{23}{5}$; $\frac{1}{2}x = 69$; $x = 69 \times 2 = 138$.

32. B. $\frac{20}{1} = \frac{240}{x}$. 20x = 240. $x = \frac{240}{20} = 12$ hours.

33. C. If x represents the original price of the jacket and y represents the discounted amount, then $0.30x = y$ and $x - y = 28$; $x - 0.30x = 28$; $0.70x = 28$; $x = \dfrac{28}{0.70} = \$40$.

34. A. The volume of a cylinder can be found by the equation $V = \pi r^2 h$. $V = 3.14 \times (3^2) \times 12$. $3.14 \times 9 \times 12 = 339.12$ cu. in.

35. C: In both equations, the coefficient of m is the rate of change. In this problem, the rate of change represents the customer's monthly cost. Therefore the customers at John's Gym pay $40 per month, and the customers at Ralph's Recreation Room pay $45 per month. Thus, John's monthly membership fee is less than Ralph's monthly membership fee.

36. C: That data points in this scatter plot form a curve. This is a nonlinear association. Therefore, choice C is correct.

Science Test

1. D. The cellular hierarchy starts with the cell, the simplest structure, and progresses to organisms, the most complex structures.

2. A: Our skin and mucus membranes are the first line of defense against potentially invading bacteria. Their purpose is to keep the bacteria from getting into the body in the first place. Any break or tear in the skin or mucus membranes can allow harmful bacteria or viruses to attack the body. Once inside, macrophages, T-cells, and lymphocytes will be summoned to attack infected body cells and the invading pathogens.

3. C. Interphase is the period when the DNA is replicated (or when the chromosomes are replicated) and is the longest part of the cell cycle.

4. B. Recessive alleles are represented by lower case letters, while dominant alleles are represented by upper case letters,

5. C. Dominant genes are always expressed when both alleles are dominant (BB) or when one is dominant and one is recessive (Bg). In this case, $\frac{3}{4}$ or 75% will have brown eyes.

6. B: Evidence used to make a scientific conclusion must be reproducible, meaning the same results would occur time and again if an experiment was repeated. The boiling point of water, for instance, always remains the same, regardless of where, when, or how many times it is measured. Evidence used to make scientific conclusions can be quantitative or qualitative, making (A) incorrect, and evidence doesn't have to be obvious to be valid, making (C) an incorrect choice. Since (A) and (C) are incorrect, (D) is also incorrect.

7. D. The nuclear division of somatic cells takes place during mitosis.

8. B: The reticular activating system (RAS) is primarily responsible for the arousal and maintenance of consciousness. The midbrain is a part of the brainstem, which has a crucial role in the regulation of autonomic functions like breathing and heart rate. The diencephalon consists of the hypothalamus and thalamus in the middle part of the brain between the cerebrum and midbrain. It plays a huge role in regulating and coordinating sensory information and hormonal secretion from the hypothalamus. The limbic system tends to the major instinctual drives like eating, sex, thirst, and aggression.

9. D. The rate at which a chemical reaction occurs does not depend on the amount of mass lost, since the law of conservation of mass (or matter) states that in a chemical reaction there is no loss of mass.

10. B. It is impossible for an *AaBb* organism to have the *aa* combination in the gametes. It is impossible for each letter to be used more than one time, so it would be impossible for the lowercase *a* to appear twice in the gametes. It would be possible, however, for *Aa* to appear in the gametes, since there is one uppercase *A* and one lowercase *a*. Gametes are the cells involved in sexual reproduction. They are germ cells.

11. A: A good hypothesis is testable and logical, and can be used to predict future events. A good hypothesis is also simple, not complex. Therefore, the correct choice is A.

12. A. A ribosome is a structure of eukaryotic cells that makes proteins.

13. C: Scientists make observations, gather data, and complete research over many years in order to compile knowledge that will provide insight into future disasters, such as earthquakes, storms, and global warming. Although science can be used to predict earthquakes and other natural disasters, there is currently no way of preventing them from occurring.

14. C: The hydrogen bonds between water molecules cause water molecules to attract each other (negative pole to positive pole. and "stick" together. This gives water a high surface tension, which allows small living organisms, such as water striders, to move across its surface. Since water is a polar molecule, it readily dissolves other polar and ionic molecules such as carbohydrates and amino acids. Polarity alone is not sufficient to make something soluble in water, however; for example, cellulose is polar but its molecular weight is so large that it is not soluble in water.

15. B: The only purpose of muscles is to produce movement through contraction.

16. B. Metals are usually solids at room temperature, while nonmetals are usually gases at room temperature.

17. D: Every month during a normal menstrual cycle, a single egg is released from the ovary and moves down the fallopian tubes toward the uterus. If sperm cells are in the reproductive tract, they will encounter and fertilize the egg in the fallopian tubes. The fertilized egg will subsequently travel the rest of the way into the uterus and implant in the uterine lining.

18. D: In order to investigate the effects of fertilizer on grass height, the student needs to have a control sample. He should only fertilize one pot so he can compare the differences in growth between the two. Measuring more frequently (A) and accurately (C) would still not allow him to make any conclusions since there is no control sample. The student is investigating the effect of fertilizer, not water (B), so both plants must be given equal amounts of water.

19. A: Smooth is not a type of connective tissue. Cartilage, adipose tissue, and blood tissue all are.

20. D. Intensive properties do not depend on the amount of matter that is present. Mass, weight, and volume do depend on the amount of matter that is present, and are considered extensive properties. Density does not depend on the amount of matter that is present, and is therefore considered an intensive property.

21. A. The trait Ll describes the genotype of the person or the traits for the genes they carry. It is heterozygous because it contains a dominant gene and a recessive gene. Tallness is the phenotype of the person or the physical expression of the genes they carry, because L for tallness is the dominant gene.

22. B. Each chromosome contains many genes, which is the basic unit of heredity. Each gene is coded by a number of DNA base pairs; the average gene contains twenty-seven thousand base pairs. A human chromosome is a single strand of DNA, which is usually tightly coiled. Human chromosomes average more than sixty million base pairs; each human chromosome contains, on average, about seven hundred genes (though some chromosomes contain more than others).

23. A: Pure water will always freeze at the same temperature: 0° Celsius, or 32° Fahrenheit. The temperature at which iron ore will melt (B) varies depending on the types of impurities that are present in the substance. The human population size (C) has been changing ever since humans first inhabited the earth. The time the sun rises (D) varies according to the time of year and the location of the observer.

24. B: The lymphatic system includes the spleen.

25. D. Smooth muscle tissue involuntarily contracts to assist the digestive tract by moving the stomach and helping with the breakdown of food.

26. C: The SA node in the right atrium generates the impulse that travels through the heart tissue and to the AV node. The AV node sits in the wall of the right atrium and coordinates atrial and ventricular contraction of the heart. The impulse then travels down to the bundle of His, the two main (left and right) branches of conduction fibers and to the Perkinje fibers which spread the impulse throughout the rest of the heart.

27. D: Langerhans cells and melanocytes both have protective functions, though melanocytes protect the skin against UVA and UVB radiation. Langerhans cells are found in the epidermis and assist lymphocytes in processing foreign antigens. Eccrine glands secrete sweat, which aids in temperature regulation and excretion of water and electrolytes. Reticular fibers make up part of the structure of the extracellular material.

28. A. The central nervous system is the main control center for the human body and is composed of the brain and spinal cord.

29. C: Afferent vessels carry fluid toward a structure; efferent vessels carry fluid away from the structure. So afferent lymph vessels carry lymph towards the node, and efferent vessels carry lymph away from the node.

30. A: Descriptive studies are usually the first form of study in a new area of scientific inquiry. Others are also forms of scientific study, but are completed after initial descriptive studies.

31. A. The circulatory system gets its name from the fact that it circulates blood and other substances throughout the body in the bloodstream. These chemicals include nutrients obtained from food, as well as oxygen, carbon dioxide and other chemicals and hormones. The digestive system breaks down food into proteins, fats and sugars that the body can use. The respiratory system exchanges oxygen and carbon dioxide between the air and the body tissues. The urinary system removes wastes from the body.

32. B: The duodenum is the first segment of the small intestine, connecting to the stomach on one end and to the ileum on the other. The ileum sits between the duodenum and the last section of small intestine, the jejunum, which then connects to the large intestine.

33. C. Isotopes are atoms of the same element with different atomic masses. Since they are of the same element, they must have equal numbers of protons. Therefore, to have different atomic masses (number of protons plus neutrons), they must have different numbers of neutrons. The number of electrons depends on the atom's ionization state; if both isotopes are electrically neutral, they will have the same number of electrons. Isotopes cannot differ in the number of nuclei; every atom has one nucleus (though that nucleus may contain numerous protons and neutrons).

34. C. The diaphragm is a large, flat muscle located at the base of the rib cage. The contractions of the diaphragm enlarge the thoracic cavity, decreasing the pressure in the lungs and drawing in air. Air is then expelled when the diaphragm relaxes. This allows the thoracic cavity to return to its former size and volume. Because it plays a role in breathing, the diaphragm is considered to be a part of the respiratory system.

35. C. One of the primary purposes of the platelets is to aggregate and form a blood clot when bleeding occurs, such as from a wound or injury. This clot blocks the opening in the damaged blood vessel and prevents further loss of blood from the body. Oxygen is carried by the red blood cells, or erythrocytes. Pathogens and other foreign materials are eliminated by the white blood cells, or leukocytes. Nutrients derived from food are carried directly in the plasma.

36. D. Chemical and electrical signals traveling through the nervous system must typically pass through multiple neurons, or nerve cells. They pass from one neuron to another across a gap called the synapse. The axon is a projection of the neuron that carries signals away from the cell body, while the dendrite receives and carries incoming signals toward the cell body. A ganglion is a mass of neurons located outside the brain.

37. B. There are three types of muscle tissue: cardiac, skeletal, and smooth. The muscles that are under voluntary control and are used for movement and locomotion are the skeletal muscles. Smooth muscle is found in the walls of the stomach, esophagus, and other organs. Cardiac muscle is similar to smooth muscle in that it is not under conscious control, but it is found only in the heart. There is no such thing as nodular muscle.

38. D. Peristalsis is the term used to describe muscular contractions that move food through the esophagus and intestines. Homeostasis is the body's maintenance of a stable internal environment. Ingestion describes the whole process of taking in nutrients, rather than any particular stage in that process. Metastasis describes the spread of cancerous cells to other tissues or organs.

39. A: Repeating a measurement several times can increase the accuracy of the measurement. Calibrating the equipment (b) will increase the precision of the measurement. None of the other choices are useful strategies to increase the accuracy of a measurement.

40. A. The region of the body below the ribcage and above the pelvis is called the *abdomen*. The thorax, also known as the chest, is the part of the body within the ribcage. The peritoneum is a membrane that surrounds the abdominal cavity, but does not describe the entire region. Likewise the umbilicus, or navel, is located in the abdomen but is not descriptive of the whole area.

41. C: Smooth muscle cells are elongated and spindle shaped. Cardiac muscle cells are cross-striated and quadrangular. Epithelial cells are tightly packed and cuboidal. This eliminates choices A, B, and D. Skeletal muscle cells are striated, cylindrical fibers with nuclei located towards the outer edges of the fibers.

42. A. The immune system plays an important role in the human body, protecting it against harmful bacteria, viruses and other foreign threats. Sometimes, however, the immune system develops a hypersensitivity, which means that it overreacts to stimuli that would otherwise be harmless. One example of hypersensitivity is an allergy; neither asthma nor cancer can be traced to a hypersensitive immune system. Fever is an epiphenomenon that may accompany many clinical situations and has no particular connection to a hypersensitive immune system.

43. D. The nervous system serves several important functions. It obtains data from the internal and external environment (in part through the sensory organs), and processes and integrates the collected information. Finally, it sends signals to activate glands and muscles to create an appropriate reaction. While the nervous system does exert some control over the production of hormones, as it does most other aspects of bodily functions, the glands that produce those hormones are not considered part of the nervous system, but rather comprise the endocrine system.

44. B. A woman is most likely to become pregnant around the time of ovulation, the part of the menstrual cycle in which a mature ovum, or egg, is released into the oviduct. This typically occurs a14 days after the start of menstruation. Because the menstrual cycle can vary in length, however, the rhythm method, or timing intercourse to avoid ovulation, is not a reliable method of avoiding pregnancy.

45. A: A hinge joint can only move in two directions. The elbow is a hinge joint. It can only bring the lower arm closer to the upper arm or move it away from the upper arm. In a ball-and-socket joint, the rounded top of one bone fits into a concave part of another bone, enabling the first bone to rotate around in this socket. This connection is slightly less stable than other types of joints in the human body and is therefore supported by a denser network of ligaments. The shoulder and hip are both examples of ball-and-socket joints.

46. D: The force of *blood pressure* motivates filtration in the kidneys. *Filtration* is the process through which the kidneys remove waste products from the body. All of the water in the blood passes through the kidneys every 45 minutes. Waste products are diverted into ducts and excreted from the body, while the healthy components of the water in blood are reabsorbed into the bloodstream. *Peristalsis* is the set of involuntary muscle movements that move food through the digestive system.

47. C. The Golgi apparatus is sometimes called the cell's "mailroom" or "shipping department." Proteins and other large molecules produced in the endoplasmic reticulum are brought to the Golgi apparatus, where they are modified and packaged for transport elsewhere in the cell. The cell's genetic material is contained in the nucleus. The cell's shape and structural integrity are due mainly to the cell membrane and the cytoskeleton. Cellular metabolic processes take place in the mitochondria.

48. A: HCG is secreted by the trophoblast, part of the early embryo, following implantation in the uterus. GnRH (gonadotropin-releasing hormone. is secreted by the hypothalamus, while LH (luteinizing hormone. and FSH (follicle-stimulating hormone. are secreted by the pituitary gland. GnRH stimulates the production of LH and FSH. LH stimulates ovulation and the production of estrogen and progesterone by the ovary in females, and testosterone production in males. FSH stimulates maturation of the ovarian follicle and estrogen production in females and sperm production in males.

49. A. The process by which a less specialized cell develops into a more specialized form is known as cellular differentiation. This process is vital to the growth and development of humans and other complex multicellular organisms. A human embryo starts as a single undifferentiated cell. It then divides and differentiates into the roughly two hundred different kinds of cells in the adult human body.

50. C: The vocal cords are located in the larynx. These elastic bands vibrate and produce sound when air passes through them. The *larynx* lies between the pharynx and the trachea. The pharynx is the section of the throat that extends from the mouth and the nasal cavities to the larynx, at which point it becomes the esophagus. The *trachea* is the tube running from the larynx down to the lungs, where it terminates in the *bronchi*. The *epiglottis* is the flap that blocks food from the lungs by descending over the trachea during a swallow.

51. C: A good experiment has only one variable, several constants, and a control. This experiment has all of these. However, this experiment lacks repetition. The student should use a group of plants—not just one—to investigate the effect of each pH on plant growth. Therefore, the correct choice is C.

52. D: Accuracy is determined by finding the range of differences between the measured values and the actual value. The smaller the differences, the greater the accuracy. The range of differences for the triple beam balance is between 0.004 – 0.016. The range of differences for the digital balance is 0.001 – 0.002. Therefore, the digital balance is more accurate. Precision is determined by finding the difference between the highest and lowest readings for each balance. The smaller the difference, the greater the precision. This range for the triple beam balance is 0.02. This range for the digital balance is 0.001. Therefore, the digital balance is also more precise.

53. A: Blood pH in mammals is chiefly regulated by the kidneys and lungs. The lungs remove nearly all of the CO_2 from the blood, preventing acidosis. Bicarbonate is adjusted by the kidneys to prevent acidosis and alkalosis. Therefore, the correct answer is A.

English and Language Usage Test

1. A. Volleyball is a team sport that follows the verb "to play," whereas individual sports like yoga follow the verb "to do."

2. B. The term "student" is general, so the relative clause is essential to the meaning of the sentence and should not be separated out by commas.

3. B. The second sentence is the clearest, since there are misplaced modifiers and verb confusion in the other sentences.

4. D. The word "every" is a singular noun and should be followed by a singular pronoun. In this case, the only singular pronoun is "her."

5. D: First the writer should narrow down all topics included to a main idea. Then s/he should identify main points supporting that main idea, decide how to sequence those main points, list all the details that support each of the main points, and then organize those details in a chosen sequential order (e.g., by association, by logical progression, from strongest to weakest, or from weakest to strongest).

6. C: "Because he was late" is the one dependent clause (a), (c) that cannot stand alone; it is introduced by the subordinating conjunction "Because" and modifies "he missed the field trip," the first independent clause, which could stand alone as a sentence. This is joined by the coordinating conjunction "and" to the second independent clause, "this caused him to fail the class." Hence there is not only one independent clause (a), (b), nor are there two dependent clauses (b), (d).

7. B: Version (a) is compound, i.e., two independent clauses (joined by a semicolon). Version (b) is complex, i.e., one independent clause ("You will have to come back tomorrow") and one dependent clause ("since you arrived past the deadline today") connected and introduced by the subordinating conjunction "since." Version (c) is simple, i.e., one independent clause, including a compound predicate ("arrived" and "will have to come back") but no dependent clause. Version (d) is compound-complex, with two independent clauses ("You arrived late" and "you must come back tomorrow") and one dependent clause ("which was after the deadline").

8. A: The meaning of *trans-* as "across" can be discerned based on vocabulary words like *transport* (carry across), *translate* and *transfer* (both meaning to bear or carry across), *transgender* (across gender), *transition* (crossing or going across), *transduce* (to convert across forms, e.g., of energy), etc. All these share the common prefix meaning of across or from one place or thing to another. One prefix meaning "change" (b) is *meta-* (e.g., metamorphosis). *Port-* as in "portable" means carry (c). A prefix meaning "different" (d) is *hetero-* (e.g., heterosexual, heterogeneous, heterocyclic, heteromorphic).

9. D: A large inscribed stone. A stele is a large, upright stone that typically has writing on it. It is used as a monument; steles were commonly used in ancient cultures in the Middle East.

10. D: It is the height of hypocrisy to acknowledge that global warming is a problem and then still tool around in a gas-guzzling car. This is the only choice that fails to maintain a formal, objective stance.

11. A: The first sentence introduces an argument against complete freedom of speech. The second sentence makes an argument in favor of it. The second sentence contradicts the first one, so the two sentences should be linked with the adverb "however." "Therefore" and "so" would be used only if the sentences supported each other.

12. D: To defame someone is to damage his or her reputation through words. To vilify is to use words in an abusive way towards someone's reputation. It is stronger and, so, makes the statement more negative. Gently mocking or embarrassing someone, while close in meaning to defaming, are weaker forms of ridicule and would not give the term a more negative connotation. Choice B bears little relation to the original word.

13. B: The key to an effective concluding statement is a concise summary of the argument's main points. Such a conclusion leaves the opponent and audience with a clear and organized understanding of the argument. The introduction of new points or a detail merely added to lighten mood would weaken the argument by straying off point at the last minute. Introducing contradictory perspectives completely would work against the argument's effectiveness.

14. C: In answer A, the comma should be a semicolon, since these are two independent clauses that are related. In answer B, there is no reason to add a comma to the phrase "quickly and cautiously." In answer D, the semicolon is used inappropriately.

15. A: Adverbs are words that modify a verb, an adjective, or another adverb. The adverb in this sentence is "happily," and it describes how Amy accepted the flowers.

16. C: The sentence is about a woman who has been held against her will for many days. It makes sense that she would plead or beg for her release. That she would throw, sympathize, or anger for her release does not.

17. B: If something that is antibacterial kills bacteria, it can't be original to it, before it, or under it. The only answer choice that makes sense is B, which is against. The antibacterial agent goes against what enables the bacteria to live.

18. C: This answer choice is the simplest and most efficient way of expressing the same ideas that are in the original sentence. The remainder of the answer choices contain redundancies, passive language, and poor sentence structure.

19. A: Answer B should be "interim," answer C should be "embellish," and answer D should be "fulcrum."

20. D: Answer D is the best choice, as it corrects the misplaced modifier error in the sentence. Max is clearly the subject of the sentence, and therefore his name needs to be the first word after the comma. Answers A and B change the meaning of the sentence. Answer C repeats the same error as the one found in the original sentence.

21. C: The subject of the sentence should be "Ben," but the noun that follows the comma at the end of the opening phrase names the subject as "the college Ben chose." This doesn't make sense, and is an example of a misplaced or dangling modifier. The subject, "the college Ben chose," agrees with the verb "was." "Harvard" is a noun, not a preposition.

22. C: A compound sentence contains two independent clauses joined with a coordinating conjunction. Answer A is a simple sentence. Answer B is a compound/complex sentence. Answer D is a complex sentence.

23. B: The colon in this sentence correctly introduces a list of items. In answer A, the semicolon should be a comma. In answer C, there should be a question mark instead of a period. In answer D, the comma should be a semicolon.

24. C: Adjacent means next to or abutting. In the case of countries, adjacent states necessarily share a border. Choices A and B are possible if two countries are next to one another, but it is not necessarily true. Distant carries the opposite meaning of adjacent.

25. B: "Terra" is a Latin root word that means "earth." An *extraterrestrial* is someone who is not born on Earth; *terrain* refers to a certain area of land.

26. A: A predicate adjective. A predicate adjective is an adjective that comes after a linking verb (such as the verb "to be") and modifies or describes the subject. In this example, "puppy" is the subject, "is" is the linking verb, and "protective" is the adjective.

27. B: paroxysm. A paroxysm is a fit or sudden attack of a disease or emotion.

28. B: To elaborate means to develop an idea more clearly. The addition of the preposition "on," used to make the verb transitive, gives a nuance to the phrase that begs the question of how one elaborates. In this case, adding detail to what is said allows the ideas to become more fully developed.

TEAS Practice Test #2

Reading

DIRECTIONS: The reading practice test you are about to take is multiple-choice with only one correct answer per question. Read each test item and circle your answer on the answer sheet below. When you have completed the practice test, you may check your answers with the answers on the answer key following the test.

Answer Sheet

1.	a	b	c	d		29.	a	b	c	d
2.	a	b	c	d		30.	a	b	c	d
3.	a	b	c	d		31.	a	b	c	d
4.	a	b	c	d		32.	a	b	c	d
5.	a	b	c	d		33.	a	b	c	d
6.	a	b	c	d		34.	a	b	c	d
7.	a	b	c	d		35.	a	b	c	d
8.	a	b	c	d		36.	a	b	c	d
9.	a	b	c	d		37.	a	b	c	d
10.	a	b	c	d		38.	a	b	c	d
11.	a	b	c	d		39.	a	b	c	d
12.	a	b	c	d		40.	a	b	c	d
13.	a	b	c	d		41.	a	b	c	d
14.	a	b	c	d		42.	a	b	c	d
15.	a	b	c	d		43.	a	b	c	d
16.	a	b	c	d		44.	a	b	c	d
17.	a	b	c	d		45.	a	b	c	d
18.	a	b	c	d		46.	a	b	c	d
19.	a	b	c	d		47.	a	b	c	d
20.	a	b	c	d		48.	a	b	c	d
21.	a	b	c	d		49.	a	b	c	d
22.	a	b	c	d		50.	a	b	c	d
23.	a	b	c	d		51.	a	b	c	d
24.	a	b	c	d		52.	a	b	c	d
25.	a	b	c	d		53.	a	b	c	d
26.	a	b	c	d						
27.	a	b	c	d						
28.	a	b	c	d						

The next four questions are based on the following passage.

It could be argued that all American war movies take as their governing paradigm that of the Western, and that we, as viewers, don't think critically enough about this fact. The virtuous hero in the white hat, the evil villain in the black hat, the community threatened by violence; these are the obvious elements of the paradigm. In addition, the hero is highly skilled at warfare, though reluctant to use it, the community is made up of morally upstanding citizens, and there is no place for violence in the community: the hero himself must leave the community he has saved once the battle is complete. This way of seeing the world has soaked into our storytelling of battle and conflict. It's hard to find a U.S.-made war movie that, for example, presents the enemy as complex and potentially fighting a legitimate cause, or that presents the hero (usually the U.S.) as anything other than supremely morally worthy. It is important to step back and think about the assumptions and frameworks that shape the stories we're exposed to; if we're careless and unquestioning, we absorb biases and world views with which we may not agree.

1. The primary purpose of this passage is to:
    a. analyze an interesting feature of American cinema.
    b. refute the Western paradigm.
    c. suggest a way that war movies could be made better.
    d. suggest that viewers think critically about underlying assumptions in the movies we watch.

2. The author claims that it is hard to find a U.S. made movie that "presents the hero (usually the U.S.) as anything other than supremely morally worthy." Does the author imply that she:
    a. believes the hero should always appear to be morally worthy.
    b. believes the hero should never appear to be morally worthy.
    c. believes the hero should be more nuanced and less unconditionally good.
    d. believes the hero is an uninteresting character.

3. Which of the following is <u>not</u> an example given by the author of an element of the Western paradigm:
    a. Hero highly skilled at warfare
    b. Evil villain in black hat
    c. Everyone riding horses
    d. Community made up of upstanding citizens

4. Which of the following is part of the world view, with which we may not agree, that the author implies we might absorb from these movies if we're careless and unquestioning:
    a. Enemies of the U.S. do not ever fight for legitimate causes.
    b. The community is morally bankrupt.
    c. The U.S. is complex.
    d. The U.S. is not skilled at warfare.

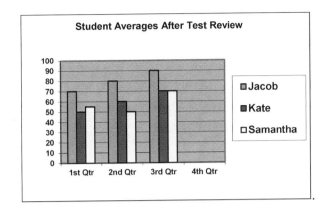

5. Using the table above, what conclusions can be made about the students' scores?
    a. The scores increased as the year progressed
    b. The girls did better than the boys on the test each quarter
    c. The test was about Math
    d. The scores were heavily impacted by the test reviews that were provided

---

The next three questions are based on the following advertisement.

Job Description:
Assistant City Attorney – City of Elm

The City of Elm is now hiring for the position of assistant City Attorney, litigation. Candidates must be members in Good Standing of the California Bar Association. Ideal candidates will have:

- at least 3 years litigation experience
- the ability to work both self-directed and as part of a team
- the ability to manage a large caseload

Competitive salary and excellent benefits offered. Position available immediately. Send completed application to:

HR Department
Attention Veronica Smith
1 City Center Plaza
Elm, California 95763

6. According to the advertisement, which of the following is true?
    a. Candidates must have three or more years litigation experience
    b. Candidates will have small caseloads
    c. Candidates must be members of the California State Bar Association
    d. The position is not currently available

7. A "competitive salary" is one that is
   a. Much less than salaries offered for comparable jobs
   b. Much greater than salaries offered for comparable jobs
   c. Similar to the average salary offered for comparable jobs
   d. Impossible to compare to the salaries offered for comparable jobs

8. It can be inferred from the advertisement that
   a. A person staffing this position may work independently and/or as part of a team.
   b. Veronica Davis will make the hiring decisions.
   c. Caseloads will start out small for new hires.
   d. A candidate could work part-time if he or she chose to.

The next three questions are based on the following passage.

The federal government regulates dietary supplements through the United States Food and Drug Administration (FDA). The regulations for dietary supplements are not the same as those for prescription or over-the-counter drugs. In general, the regulations for dietary supplements are less strict.

To begin with, a manufacturer does not have to prove the safety and effectiveness of a dietary supplement before it is marketed. A manufacturer is permitted to say that a dietary supplement addresses a nutrient deficiency, supports health, or is linked to a particular body function (such as immunity), if there is research to support the claim. Such a claim must be followed by the words "This statement has not been evaluated by the Food and Drug Administration. This product is not intended to diagnose, treat, cure, or prevent any disease."

Also, manufacturers are expected to follow certain good manufacturing practices (GMPs) to ensure that dietary supplements are processed consistently and meet quality standards. Requirements for GMPs went into effect in 2008 for large manufacturers and are being phased in for small manufacturers through 2010.

Once a dietary supplement is on the market, the FDA monitors safety and product information, such as label claims and package inserts. If it finds a product to be unsafe, it can take action against the manufacturer and/or distributor and may issue a warning or require that the product be removed from the marketplace. The Federal Trade Commission (FTC) is responsible for regulating product advertising; it requires that all information be truthful and not misleading.

The federal government has taken legal action against a number of dietary supplement promoters or Web sites that promote or sell dietary supplements because they have made false or deceptive statements about their products or because marketed products have proven to be unsafe.

9. What is the main idea of the passage?
   a. Manufacturers of dietary supplements have to follow good manufacturing practices.
   b. The FDA has a special program for regulating dietary supplements.
   c. The federal government prosecutes those who mislead the general public.
   d. The FDA is part of the federal government.

10. Which statement is *not* a detail from the passage?
  a. Promoters of dietary supplements can make any claims that are supported by research.
  b. GMP requirements for large manufacturers went into effect in 2008.
  c. Product advertising is regulated by the FTc.
  d. The FDA does not monitor products after they enter the market.

11. What is the meaning of the word *deceptive* as it is used in the fifth paragraph?
  a. misleading
  b. malicious
  c. illegal
  d. irritating

12. Which of the following choices introduces a specific claim and distinguishes it from counterclaims?
  a. Is texting while driving really a critical safety issue? Are all kinds of distracted driving created equal? What can be said about the nature of distracted driving among teenagers?
  b. It's true that distracted driving is dangerous. There may be nothing more dangerous than texting while driving. Texting while driving has resulted in more than 15,000 deaths and over 200,000 injuries. The majority of texting drivers are teens, although other age groups have been implicated.
  c. Texting while driving is one of the key issues facing young people today: it's a fact that texting drivers have killed over 16,000 people between 2002 and 2007. While some people claim that any kind of distracted driving is dangerous, texting beats them all by keeping attention away from the road.
  d. Driving and texting have gone hand in hand ever since the first teen decided that he needed to let his friends know what he was thinking right then and there. Government offices have kept tabs on distracted drivers, and the numbers are staggering. The years of the study were from 2002 to 2007.

13. Which of the following would be the best source to begin developing a position about civil rights for an oral debate?
  a. A blog created by a proponent of civil rights.
  b. An interview with someone who took part in a civil rights march.
  c. A history textbook detailing civil rights.
  d. A speech by a famous civil rights leader.

14. Among the following structural patterns in a paragraph, which does a writer use to show readers something instead of telling them something?
  a. Division
  b. Narration
  c. Definition
  d. Description

A librarian is approached by a student who wants to do an Internet search for Thomas Jefferson but does not know how. The student has been assigned to read a biography of Jefferson and then write a report on his life, which is due in ten days.

15. What is the librarian's best course of action in this situation?
    a. The librarian shows the student how to do an Internet search using Google
    b. Since the assignment is to read a biography, the librarian directs the student to the biography section of the library rather than to the Internet. She helps the student select a biography at his reading level
    c. The librarian directs the student to database that will quickly provide a list of resources and articles pertaining to Thomas Jefferson
    d. The librarian searches her computerized records, decides that none of the biographies in her school library are appropriate for this student, and initiates an inter-library loan. The borrowed biography will take about two weeks to arrive

---

16. Which of the following sentences uses the word "smart" with a negative connotation, rather than a positive connotation or simply the word's denotation?
    a. Eliot's teacher said he was not quite gifted, but too smart for a general class.
    b. Eliot was smart to have studied the day before the test; he got a good grade.
    c. Eliot was identified by his teacher as one of the smart students in her classes.
    d. Eliot got into trouble when he gave a smart answer to his teacher's question.

In three pieces of informational writing, sample 1's author provides evidence tangential to his argument. Sample 2's author cites anecdotal evidence that is inaccurate. Sample 3's author cites accurate, directly related evidence, but it is an isolated example uncorroborated by any other sources.

17. Which choice correctly matches these samples with incompletely met criteria?
    a. Sample 1's evidence is not sufficient; sample 2's is not relevant; sample 3's is not factual.
    b. Sample 1's evidence is not factual; sample 2's is not sufficient; sample 3's is not relevant.
    c. Sample 1's evidence is not relevant; sample 2's is not factual; sample 3's is not sufficient.
    d. The evidence of samples 1 and 3 is insufficient; sample 2's evidence is factual but irrelevant.

---

18. Using the dictionary guide words above, which of the following words is most likely to appear on the *following* page of the dictionary?
    a. deleterious
    b. dehydrate
    c. delay
    d. deity

19. For evaluating the credibility of a source when doing research, which of these is true?
    a. The author's reputation is more important than whether s/he cites sources.
    b. The source should always be as recent as possible, regardless of the subject.
    c. The author's point of view and/or purpose is not germane to the credibility.
    d. The kinds of sources various audiences value influence credibility for them.

The next three questions are based on the following passage.

The loss of barrier islands through erosion poses a serious challenge to many communities along the Atlantic and Gulf Coasts. Along with marshes and wetlands, these islands protect coastal towns from major storms. In the past seventy years, Louisiana alone has lost almost 2,000 square miles of coastal land to hurricanes and flooding. More than 100 square miles of wetlands protecting the city of New Orleans were wiped out by a single storm, Hurricane Katrina. Due to this exposure of coastal communities, recent hurricane seasons have proven the most expensive on record: annual losses since 2005 have been estimated in the hundreds of billions of dollars. This unfortunate trend is likely to continue, since meteorological research shows that the Atlantic basin is in an active storm period that could continue for decades.

20. Which of the following statements offers a supporting argument for the passage's claim that many coastal islands are eroding?
    a. Recent hurricane seasons have been expensive.
    b. The Atlantic Basin is entering an active period.
    c. Louisiana has lost 2,000 square miles of coastal land.
    d. Barrier islands are the first line of defense against coastal storms.

21. The passage describes recent hurricane seasons as the most expensive on record. Which of the following statements gives the implied reason for this increased expense?
    a. Hurricane Katrina was an extremely violent storm.
    b. Valuable buildings were destroyed in New Orleans.
    c. The Atlantic Basin is entering an active period.
    d. Destruction of barrier islands and coastal wetlands has left the mainland exposed.

22. Which of the following choices represents the best label for this passage?
    a. definition essay
    b. cause/effect essay
    c. comparison essay
    d. persuasive essay

The following is an excerpt of an article published by The New York Times *announcing the assassination of Abraham Lincoln. Use the following article to answer the next five questions.*

AWFUL EVENT

President Lincoln Shot by an Assassin

The Deed Done at Ford's Theatre Last Night

THE ACT OF A DESPERATE REBEL

The President Still Alive at Last Accounts

No Hopes Entertained of His Recovery

Attempted Assassination of Secretary Seward

DETAILS OF THE DREADFUL TRAGEDY.

Official

War Department, Washington April 15, 1:30 A.M. - Maj. Gen. Dis.: This evening at about 9:30 P.M. at Ford's Theatre, the President, while sitting in his private box with Mrs. Lincoln, Mr. Harris, and Major Rathburn, was shot by an assassin, who suddenly entered the box and appeared behind the President. The assassin then leaped upon the stage, brandishing a large dagger or knife, and made his escape in the rear of the theatre.

The pistol ball entered the back of the President's head and penetrated nearly through the head. The wound is <u>mortal</u>. The President has been insensible ever since it was inflicted, and is now dying.

About the same hour an assassin, whether the same or not, entered Mr. Sewards' apartments, and under the pretense of having a prescription, was shown to the Secretary's sick chamber. The assassin immediately rushed to the bed, and inflicted two or three stabs on the throat and two on the face. It is hoped the wounds may not be mortal. My apprehension is that they will prove fatal.

The nurse alarmed Mr. Frederick Seward, who was in an adjoining room, and hastened to the door of his father's room, when he met the assassin, who inflicted upon him one or more dangerous wounds. The recovery of Frederick Seward is doubtful.

It is not probable that the President will live throughout the night.

Gen. Grant and wife were advertised to be at the theatre this evening, but he started to Burlington at 6 o'clock this evening. At a Cabinet meeting at which Gen. Grant was present, the subject of the state of the country and the prospect of a speedy peace was discussed. The President was very cheerful and hopeful, and spoke very kindly of Gen. Lee and others of the Confederacy, and of the establishment of government in Virginia.

All the members of the Cabinet except Mr. Seward are now in attendance upon the President. I have seen Mr. Seward, but he and Frederick were both unconscious.

Edwin M. Stanton, Secretary of War.

23. The underlined word <u>mortal</u> means
    a. recuperative.
    b. painful.
    c. fatal.
    d. risky.

24. What is a likely purpose for including so many headlines at the start of the article?
    a. to quickly convey the most important information about a significant event
    b. to sensationalize a front-page news story
    c. to incite panic in readers
    d. to fill empty space on the page

25. Who is the author of this article?
    a. The New York Times
    b. Edwin M. Stanton
    c. Frederick Seward
    d. Major Rathburn

26. What is the best summary of this article?
    a. The assassin who tried to kill President Lincoln and Secretary Seward escaped into the night. After having fired his pistol at the president, he barely eluded authorities and hurried to Seward's residence. There, he stabbed both the secretary and his son, Frederick Seward.
    b. A single assassin went on a rampage tonight, starting at Ford's Theater and absconding into the night. He currently remains at large.
    c. President Lincoln was shot by an assassin at Ford's Theater; the president is not expected to survive. Secretary Seward and his son were also attacked by an assassin at their home this evening. They remain unconscious, and their chances of survival are questionable. General Grant was scheduled to be at the theater, but changed his plans and was not harmed by the evening's events.
    d. General Grant is poised to take over the role of the presidency should President Lincoln die from wounds inflicted upon him at Ford's Theater. Grant was present at a recent Cabinet meeting, where Lincoln expressed hope for the future and spoke kind words about General Lee and the Confederacy.

27. What is implied by the following sentence?

It is hoped the wounds may not be mortal. My apprehension is that they will prove fatal.

    a. Those involved with the events are hopeful for a positive outcome.
    b. There is no hope that Seward or Lincoln will recover from their wounds.
    c. The writer is pessimistic about whether Seward will recover from his wounds.
    d. The writer is doubtful about the legitimacy of accounts regarding the night's events.

The next four questions are based on the following passage.

Magnesium is an important nutrient that supports immune system functioning and helps protect the body against cardiovascular diseases. Symptoms of magnesium deficiency rarely surface among populations in developed countries, but concern is growing that many people may not have sufficient body stores of this metal. Surveys show that most Americans do not receive a minimum daily requirement of magnesium in their diets.

Magnesium is absorbed from foods by the intestines, before the circulatory system transports it to the body's tissues. Less than one-half of ingested magnesium normally is taken up in this way. Health issues affecting the digestive tract may impair magnesium absorbance. For example, gastrointestinal disorders such as Crohn's disease can limit magnesium uptake. The kidneys normally limit urinary excretion of magnesium, a function that can help make up for low dietary intake. However, alcohol abuse and certain medications can affect this balance and thereby lead to magnesium depletion.

Symptoms of magnesium deficiency include vomiting, fatigue, and loss of appetite. More severe cases can include symptoms such as muscular cramps, seizures, and coronary abnormalities. Magnesium insufficiency also can affect the body's ability to absorb other cations, including calcium and potassium, and can lead to other health complications. Good sources of dietary magnesium include leafy green vegetables, potatoes, nuts, and seeds.

28. Which of the following statements is true?
    a. People with magnesium deficiency commonly exhibit fatigue and loss of appetite.
    b. People with magnesium deficiencies are often asymptomatic.
    c. Severe magnesium deficiency may lead to Crohn's disease.
    d. Magnesium is not absorbed by the digestive tract.

29. Which of the following labels best describes the previous passage?
    a. comparison essay
    b. definition essay
    c. cause and effect essay
    d. persuasive essay

30. According to the passage, alcohol abuse can lead to which of the following problems?
    a. poor magnesium absorption.
    b. an impairment of kidney function.
    c. compromise of the immune system.
    d. gastrointestinal disorders.

31. The word "cation" is closest in meaning to:
    a. element
    b. nutrient similar to magnesium
    c. symptom of deficiency
    d. nutritional supplement

32. To evaluate the credibility of research sources, which of the following is a valid consideration?
    a. It is credible if published in a peer-reviewed scholarly journal.
    b. It is never credible if it is a source which was published online.
    c. It is not found to be more credible through author affiliations.
    d. It is immaterial to credibility how many times a source is cited.

Gemma is planning her vacation and has been hoping for several years to travel to Hawaii. She only has one week to visit, though, so she has to make the most of her trip. Her goal is to see as much as possible in a short period of time, while also giving herself a chance to relax and enjoy the experience.

33. Based on this information, which of the following travel guides will be best for her?
    a. *Exploring the Hawaiian Islands: The Best Waterfalls on the Big Island and Maui*
    b. *Na Pali: The Two-Day Hike That Changes Everything*
    c. *Pineapples, Taro, and Roasted Pigs: A Dining Guide to Hawaii*
    d. *The Top Ten: Beaches, Restaurants, and Sightseeing in Honolulu and on Oahu*

You are preparing for a class discussion on a local issue: should the town acquire a wetland in order to protect it? You have access to two sources of information. Evaluate the views in both sources.

1) A retired physics professor, being interviewed on a morning news show, mentions: "It's obvious that our town needs to buy this land. We have to protect what we have from greedy developers who only want to turn a profit."

2) An article written by an ecologist on a well-known news site notes: "It is in our best interest to purchase this land. Wetlands are disappearing and there are not enough private donors to help with their protection."

34. Which source provides the best material for your assignment?
    a. It may be true that some businesses profit from buying up wetlands; however, the important point is that wetlands are disappearing. An ecologist noted that there are not enough private donors to buy these places.
    b. Greedy businesses are at the heart of the problem: they simply want to buy up cheap land to build and make money. They don't care about destroying our natural treasures. The physics professor noted that our town needs to buy this land.
    c. It's clear that wetlands are endangered; they are going to disappear unless we do something about it. We should get private donors to buy the land. An ecologist noted that wetlands are in danger.
    d. Businesses are part of the wetland problem. Without developers to buy them up, the town would not need to purchase the land to protect it. A physics professor noted that the wetland problem is related to greed.

---

35. Although Cora's parents were willing to humor her <u>fervid</u> interest in the new boy band up to a point, they felt that things had gone too far when she insisted on painting her ceiling with a mural of her favorite band member.

Which of the following is the definition for the underlined word in the sentence above?
    a. charming
    b. excessive
    c. passionate
    d. covetous

The next two questions are based on the chart below.

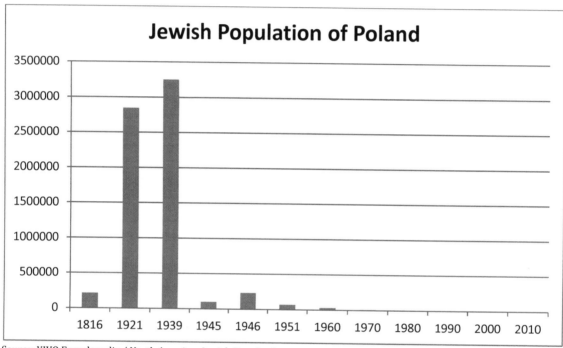

Source: YIVO Encyclopedia / North American Jewish Data Bank

36. As a result of Jewish people leaving Russia and Ukraine, the Jewish population of Poland increased dramatically. According to the chart, during which time span is this most likely to have occurred?
    a. 1816-1921
    b. 1939-1945
    c. 1945-1946
    d. 1951-1960

37. During World War II, and the years leading up to it, the Jewish population of Poland declined rapidly. Following the war, however, there was a brief period of population increase as Polish Jews returned home. According to the chart, when is this most likely to have occurred?
    a. 1939-1945
    b. 1945-1946
    c. 1946-1951
    d. 1951-1960

The next two questions are based on the information below.

Vegan and Lovin' It: Making the Transition to a Vegan Diet

Table of Contents
I. Better-for-the Planet Breads
    A. Yeast Breads
    B. Breakfast Breads and Coffee Cakes
    C. Muffins and Scones
    D. Biscuits, Pancakes and French Toast
II. Exciting Salads
    A. Salads on the Side
    B. Salads as a Meal
III. Savory Side Dishes
    A. Rice
    B. Potatoes
    C. Light Soups
    D. Veggie Delight
IV. Elegant, Easy Entrees
    A. Pasta
    B. Casseroles
    C. Hearty Soups and Stews
    D. Pizzas
    E. Slow Cooker Meals
V. Delicious Desserts and Drinks
    A. Cookies, Bars
    B. Cakes, Pies, and Tarts
    C. Ice "Cream"
    D. Smoothies
VI. Tips for Entertaining
    A. Satisfying a Crowd
    B. Recommended menus

38. Sarah is hosting a brunch for a baby shower, and she knows that several of the guests are strict vegans. She wants to make sure she prepares certain foods correctly to ensure all her guests have something to eat. In particular, she is looking for recipes for banana bread and blueberry muffins. Which chapter of the cookbook should she consult?
    a. Chapter I
    b. Chapter II
    c. Chapter IV
    d. Chapter V

39. Sarah also wants to offer her vegan guests a slightly more filling option such as a light soup with some biscuits. Which two chapters of the cookbook should she consult?
    a. Chapter II and Chapter III
    b. Chapter I and Chapter III
    c. Chapter II and Chapter IV
    d. Chapter V and Chapter VI

Announcement to all incoming students of Chatham College:

Due to the large number of expected students, registration for fall classes is being organized alphabetically by the student's last name. Please follow the guide below to register. Students with more than one last name, or with a hyphenated last name, should use the first letter of the first last name for registration.

Our online registration system is designed to accommodate this alphabetical arrangement. **Do not** try to register on a different date or at a different time. Doing so will result in your registration being rejected and could result in a failure to enter necessary courses.

Monday, 10 AM-12 PM and 5-7 PM: Letters A through G
Monday, 1-3 PM and 8-10 PM: Letters H-N
Tuesday, 10 AM-12 PM and 5-7 PM: Letters O-S
Tuesday, 1-3 PM and 8-10 PM: Letters T-Z

40. Julie Walker-Mayfield plans to register for fall classes at Chatham College. She works during the day and doesn't get off work until 5:30 PM. She also has no internet access at work and will have to register for classes once she gets home. Taking into account her personal schedule and the registration schedule provided by the college, when will she be able go online to enter the registration system and select her classes?
   a. Monday, 10 AM-12 PM
   b. Monday, 5-7 PM
   c. Tuesday, 5-7 PM
   d. Tuesday, 8-10 PM

The next four questions are based on the passage below.

Harriet Tubman was a runaway slave from Maryland who became known as the "Moses of her people." Over the course of 10 years, and at great personal risk, she led hundreds of slaves to freedom along the Underground Railroad, a secret network of safe houses where runaway slaves could stay on their journey north to freedom. She later became a leader in the abolitionist movement, and during the Civil War she was a spy for the federal forces in South Carolina as well as a nurse.

Harriet Tubman's name at birth was Araminta Ross. She was one of 11 children of Harriet and Benjamin Ross born into slavery in Dorchester County, Maryland. As a child, Ross was "hired out" by her master as a nursemaid for a small baby. Ross had to stay awake all night so that the baby wouldn't cry and wake the mother. If Ross fell asleep, the baby's mother whipped her. From a very young age, Ross was determined to gain her freedom.

As a slave, Araminta Ross was scarred for life when she refused to help in the punishment of another young slave. A young man had gone to the store without permission, and when he returned, the overseer wanted to whip him. He asked Ross to help but she refused. When the young man started to run away, the overseer picked up a heavy iron weight and threw it at him. He missed the young man and hit Ross instead. The weight nearly crushed her skull and left a deep scar. She was unconscious for days, and suffered from seizures for the rest of her life.

In 1844, Ross married a free black named John Tubman and took his last name. She also changed her first name, taking her mother's name, Harriet. In 1849, worried that she and the other slaves on the plantation were going to be sold, Tubman decided to run away. Her husband refused to go with her, so she set out with her two brothers, and followed the North Star in the sky to guide her north to freedom. Her brothers became frightened and turned back, but she continued on and reached Philadelphia. There she found work as a household servant and saved her money so she could return to help others escape.

41. This passage is mainly about
    a. slaves in the Civil War.
    b. how slaves escaped along the Underground Railroad.
    c. Harriet Tubman's role as an abolitionist leader.
    d. Harriet Tubman's life as a slave.

42. The author of the passage describes Harriet Tubman's life as a slave to show
    a. why she wanted to escape slavery.
    b. why she was a spy during the Civil War.
    c. why she suffered from seizures.
    d. how she loved babies.

43. How is this passage structured?
    a. cause and effect
    b. problem and solution
    c. chronological order
    d. compare and contrast

44. How did Araminta Ross come to be known as Harriet Tubman?
    a. She took her husband's last name and changed her first name to her mother's name.
    b. She was named after the plantation owner's wife.
    c. She changed her name because she was wanted as an Underground Railroad runner.
    d. She changed her name to remain anonymous as a Civil War spy.

45. Mirella has recently become an ovo-lacto vegetarian, which means that she does not eat any kind of animal flesh but that she does eat eggs and dairy products. In fact, she prefers to consume either eggs or dairy products at every meal to ensure a good intake of protein. Additionally, Mirella has an allergy to wheat products, so she avoids any kind of bread. Which of the following menu items fulfills her dietary requirements?
    a. Tofu-mushroom-spinach lasagna
    b. Veggie burger on a whole-grain bun
    c. Salmon with cream sauce
    d. Stuffed baked potato with vegetable soup

The next three questions are based on the information below.

<u>The Dewey Decimal Classes</u>

000 Computer science, information, and general works
100 Philosophy and psychology
200 Religion
300 Social sciences
400 Languages
500 Science and mathematics
600 Technical and applied science
700 Arts and recreation
800 Literature
900 History, geography, and biography

46. Jensen has been assigned a project on ancient Greece, but the project terms are general. This means that he can select any topic of interest to him from Ancient Greece and focus his project around this. Jenson is overwhelmed and does not even know where to begin. What section of the library should he check first for general information about ancient Greece?
    a. 100
    b. 200
    c. 400
    d. 900

47. During his study, Jenson finds himself increasingly drawn to information about the theaters of ancient Greece and particularly to the plays that the Greeks performed. What section of the library should he check next for more resources on the written plays that have survived from ancient Greece?
    a. 200
    b. 600
    c. 700
    d. 800

48. Jenson also discovers that the meaning behind many of the plays was closely related to the polytheistic beliefs that were practiced in ancient Greece. What section of the library should he check for more information about Greek polytheism?
    a. 100
    b. 200
    c. 300
    d. 900

49. Irmengard loved spending time with her great-aunt, but she occasionally had to roll her eyes at what she considered to be Aunt Fredericka's <u>antediluvian</u> views about dating and relationships.

Which of the following is the definition for the underlined word in the sentence above?
    a. outdated
    b. confusing
    c eager
    d. hostile

A student comes to the library and you observe him wandering confusedly in the library's section of science books.

50. What is the first thing you should do to help him?
    a. Ask the student what his assignment is and what kind of books he is looking for
    b. Tell the student that books are shelved by the author's last name and let him have the opportunity to use this information to find the books he is looking for
    c. Find an opportunity later on to ask his teacher what the assignment is so that if he has difficulty locating materials the next time he comes to the library, you can help him
    d. Send another student from his class over to help him, as they both have the same assignment

---

What Are the Key Facts about Seasonal Flu Vaccine?
Center for Disease Control and Prevention (CDC)

The single best way to protect against the flu is to get vaccinated each year.

About 2 weeks after vaccination, antibodies that provide protection against influenza virus infection develop in the body.

Yearly flu vaccination should begin in September or as soon as vaccine is available and continue throughout the influenza season, into December, January, and beyond. This is because the timing and duration of influenza seasons vary. While influenza outbreaks can happen as early as October, most of the time influenza activity peaks in January or later.

In general, anyone who wants to reduce their chances of getting the flu can get vaccinated. However, it is recommended by ACIP that certain people should get vaccinated each year. They are either people who are at high risk of having serious flu complications or people who live with or care for those at high risk for serious complications. During flu seasons when vaccine supplies are limited or delayed, ACIP makes recommendations regarding priority groups for vaccination.

People who should get vaccinated each year are:
- Children aged 6 months up to their 19th birthday
- Pregnant women
- People 50 years of age and older
- People of any age with certain chronic medical conditions
- People who live in nursing homes and other long-term care facilities
- People who live with or care for those at high risk for complications from flu, including:
  - Health care workers
  - Household contacts of persons at high risk for complications from the flu
  - Household contacts and out of home caregivers of children less than 6 months of age (these children are too young to be vaccinated)

51. It is December, and you have not yet had a flu vaccine. What should you do if you are among the people for whom a vaccine is recommended?
    a. Call your doctor for an appointment and get the vaccine.
    b. Avoid other people as much as possible.
    c. Wait until next year and get a double dose.
    d. Contact your local public health board to inform them.

The next two questions are based on the following passage.

Students may take classes in a wide variety of subjects for fun or self-improvement. Some classes provide students with training in useful life skills such as cooking or personal finance. Other classes provide instruction intended for recreational purposes, with topics such as photography, pottery, or painting. Classes may consist of large or small groups, or they may involve one-on-one instruction in subjects like singing or playing a musical instrument. Classes taught by self-enrichment teachers seldom lead to a degree, and attendance in these classes is voluntary. Although often taught in non-academic settings, these classes' topics may include academic subjects such as literature, foreign languages, and history. Despite their informal nature, these courses can provide students with useful work-related skills such as knowledge of computers or foreign languages; these skills make students more attractive to potential employers.

52. Which of the following statements represents the central idea of this passage?
    a. Self-improvement classes teach work-related skills.
    b. Attendance is voluntary for self-improvement classes.
    c. Many different kinds of self-improvement classes are available.
    d. Cooking is one type of self-improvement classes.

53. Which of the following statements is true?
    a. All self-improvement classes offer training in recreational subject areas.
    b. Self-improvement classes usually are taught in non-academic settings.
    c. Some informal classes teach useful work-related skills.
    d. In order to learn a foreign language, a student must enroll in a formal, degree-granting program.

Mathematics

DIRECTIONS: The mathematics practice test you are about to take is multiple-choice with only one correct answer per question. Read each test item and circle your answer on the answer sheet below. When you have completed the practice test, you may check your answers with the answers on the answer key following the test.

Answer Sheet

1.	a	b	c	d		20.	a	b	c	d
2.	a	b	c	d		21.	a	b	c	d
3.	a	b	c	d		22.	a	b	c	d
4.	a	b	c	d		23.	a	b	c	d
5.	a	b	c	d		24.	a	b	c	d
6.	a	b	c	d		25.	a	b	c	d
7.	a	b	c	d		26.	a	b	c	d
8.	a	b	c	d		27.	a	b	c	d
9.	a	b	c	d		28.	a	b	c	d
10.	a	b	c	d		29.	a	b	c	d
11.	a	b	c	d		30.	a	b	c	d
12.	a	b	c	d		31.	a	b	c	d
13.	a	b	c	d		32.	a	b	c	d
14.	a	b	c	d		33.	a	b	c	d
15.	a	b	c	d		34.	a	b	c	d
16.	a	b	c	d		35.	a	b	c	d
17.	a	b	c	d		36.	a	b	c	d
18.	a	b	c	d						
19.	a	b	c	d						

1. A man decided to buy new furniture from Futuristic Furniture for $2600. Futuristic Furniture gave the man two choices: pay the entire amount in one payment with cash, or pay $1000 as a down payment and $120 per month for two full years in the financing plan. If the man chooses the financing plan, how much more would he pay?
   a. $1480 more
   b. $1280 more
   c. $1600 more
   d. $2480 more

2. What is the value of r in the following equation?

$29 + r = 420$

   a. $r = \dfrac{29}{420}$

   b. $r = \dfrac{420}{29}$

   c. $r = 391$

   d. $r = 449$

3. If 35% of a paycheck was deducted for taxes and 4% for insurance, what is the total percent taken out of the paycheck?
   a. 20%
   b. 31%
   c. 39%
   d. 42%

4. Kyle has $950 in savings and wishes to donate one-fifth of it to 8 local charities. He estimates that he will donate around $30 to each charity. Which of the following correctly describes the reasonableness of his estimate?
   a. It is reasonable because $240 is one-fifth of $900
   b. It is reasonable because $240 is less than one-fifth of $1,000
   c. It is not reasonable because $240 is more than one-fifth of $1,000
   d. It is not reasonable because $240 is one-fifth of $1,000

5. A woman wants to stack two small bookcases beneath a window that is $26\frac{1}{2}$ inches from the floor. The larger bookcase is $14\frac{1}{2}$ inches tall. The other bookcase is $8\frac{3}{4}$ inches tall. How tall will the two bookcases be when they are stacked together?

    a. 12 inches tall

    b. $23\frac{1}{4}$ inches tall

    c. $35\frac{1}{4}$ inches tall

    d. 41 inches tall

---

6. Juan wishes to compare the percentages of time he spends on different tasks during the workday. Which of the following representations is the most appropriate choice for displaying the data?
    a. Line plot
    b. Bar graph
    c. Line graph
    d. Circle graph

---

7. Which of the following describes a real-world situation that could be modeled by $12 + 2x = 10 + 5x$?
    a. Courtney charges a \$12 fee plus \$2 per hour to babysit. Kendra charges a \$10 fee plus \$5 per hour. Write an equation to find the number of hours for which the two charges are equal.

    b. Courtney charges a \$2 fee plus \$12 per hour to babysit. Kendra charges a \$5 fee plus \$10 per hour. Write an equation to find the number of hours for which the two charges are equal.

    c. Courtney charges a \$12 fee plus \$2 to babysit. Kendra charges a \$10 fee plus \$5 to babysit. Write an equation to find the number of hours for which the two charges are equal.

    d. Courtney charges \$10 plus \$2 per hour to babysit. Kendra charges \$12 plus \$5 per hour. Write an equation to find the number of hours for which the two charges are equal.

---

8. Adrian measures the circumference of a circular picture frame, with a radius of 3 inches. Which of the following is the best estimate for the circumference of the frame?
    a. 12 inches
    b. 16 inches
    c. 18 inches
    d. 24 inches

---

9. What is the simplest way to write the following expression?
    $5x - 2y + 4x + y$
    a. $9x - y$
    b. $9x - 3y$
    c. $9x + 3y$
    d. $x ; y$

10. A ball has a diameter of 7 inches. Which of the following best represents the volume?
    a. 165.7 in^3
    b. 179.6 in^3
    c. 184.5 in^3
    d. 192.3 in^3

---

11. Which of the following is listed in order from *greatest to least*?
    a. $\frac{4}{5}, \frac{7}{8}, \frac{1}{2}, -8, -3$

    b. $\frac{7}{8}, \frac{4}{5}, \frac{1}{2}, -3, -8$

    c. $\frac{4}{5}, \frac{1}{2}, \frac{7}{8}, -3, -8$

    d. $\frac{7}{8}, \frac{4}{5}, \frac{1}{2}, -8, -3$

---

12. To begin making her soup, Jennifer added four containers of chicken broth with 1 liter of water into the pot. Each container of chicken broth contains 410 milliliters. How much liquid is in the pot?
    a. 1.64 liters
    b. 2.64 liters
    c. 5.44 liters
    d. 6.12 liters

---

13. The ratio of employee wages and benefits to all other operational costs of a business is 2:3. If a business's operating expenses are $130,000 per month, how much money does the company spend on employee wages and benefits?
    a. $43,333.33
    b. $86,666.67
    c. $52,000.00
    d. $78,000.00

---

14. Which of the following fractions is halfway between $\frac{2}{5}$ and $\frac{4}{9}$?
    a. $\frac{2}{3}$

    b. $\frac{2}{20}$

    c. $\frac{17}{40}$

    d. $\frac{19}{45}$

---

15. If 1" on a map represents 60 ft, how many yards apart are two points if the distance between the points on the map is 10"?
    a. 1800
    b. 600
    c. 200
    d. 2

16. Which of the following is equivalent to $4 + 12 \div 4 + 8 \times 3$?
    a. 24
    b. 12
    c. 36
    d. 31

Kendra uses the pie chart below to represent the allocation of her annual income. Her annual income is $40,000.

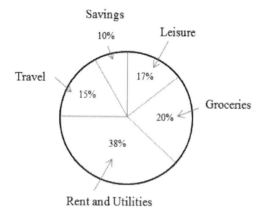

17. Which of the following statements is true?
    a. The amount of money she spends on travel and savings is more than $11,000.
    b. The amount of money she spends on rent and utilities is approximately $15,000.
    c. The amount of money she spends on groceries and savings is more than $13,000.
    d. The amount of money she spends on leisure is less than $5,000.

18. A certain exam has 30 questions. A student gets 1 point for each question he gets right and loses half a point for a question he answers incorrectly; he neither gains nor loses any points for a question left blank. If C is the number of questions a student gets right and B is the number of questions he leaves blank, which of the following represents his score on the exam?

a. $C - \frac{1}{2}B$

b. $C - \frac{1}{2}(30 - B)$

c. $C - \frac{1}{2}(30 - B - C)$

d. $(30 - C) - \frac{1}{2}(30 - B)$

---

19. In the winter of 2006, 35.6 inches of snow fell in Chicago, IL. The following winter, 60.3 inches of snowfall fell in Chicago. What was the percent increase of snowfall in Chicago between those two winters?

a. 69.4%

b. 59.0%

c. 41.0%

d. 24.7%

---

20. A taxi service charges $5.50 for the first $\frac{1}{5}$ of a mile, $1.50 for each additional $\frac{1}{5}$ of a mile, and 20¢ per minute of waiting time. Joan took a cab from her place to a flower shop 8 miles away, where she bought a bouquet, then another 3.6 miles to her mother's place. The driver had to wait 9 minutes while she bought the bouquet. What was the fare?

a. $20

b. $120.20

c. $92.80

d. $91

---

21. A commuter survey counts the people riding in cars on a highway in the morning. Each car contains only one man, only one woman, or both one man and one woman. Out of 25 cars, 13 contain a woman and 20 contain a man. How many contain both a man and a woman?

a. 4

b. 7

c. 8

d. 13

---

22. Prizes are to be awarded to the best pupils in each class of an elementary school. The number of students in each grade is shown in the table, and the school principal wants the number of prizes awarded in each grade to be proportional to the number of students. If there are twenty prizes, how many should go to fifth grade students?

Grade	1	2	3	4	5
Students	35	38	38	33	36

    a. 5
    b. 4
    c. 7
    d. 3

23. When the sampling distribution of means is plotted, which of the following is true?
    a. The distribution is approximately normal.
    b. The distribution is positively skewed.
    c. The distribution is negatively skewed.
    d. There is no predictive shape to the distribution.

24. A triangle has dimensions of 9 cm, 4 cm, and 7 cm. The triangle is reduced by a scale factor of $\frac{3}{4}$. Which of the following represents the dimensions of the dilated triangle?
    a. 8.25 cm, 3.25 cm, 6.25 cm
    b. 4.5 cm, 2 cm, 3.5 cm
    c. 6.75 cm, 3 cm, 5.25 cm
    d. 4.95 cm, 2.2 cm, 3.85 cm

25. The cost, in dollars, of shipping x computers to California for sale is 3000 + 100x. The amount received when selling these computers is 400x dollars. What is the least number of computers that must be shipped and sold so that the amount received is at least equal to the shipping cost?
    a. 10
    b. 15
    c. 20
    d. 25

26. Bob decides to go into business selling lemonade. He buys a wooden stand for $45 and sets it up outside his house. He figures that the cost of lemons, sugar, and paper cups for each glass of lemonade sold will be 10¢. Which of these expressions describes his cost for making _g_ glasses of lemonade?
    a. $45 + $0.1 × g
    b. $44.90 × g
    c. $44.90 × g + 10¢
    d. $90

27. What is the area of the shaded region in the figure shown below?

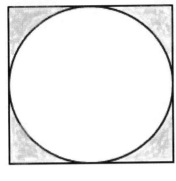

30 cm

30 cm

a. 177 cm^2
b. 181 cm^2
c. 187 cm^2
d. 193 cm^2

---

28. Sally wants to buy a used truck for her delivery business. Truck A is priced at $450 and gets 25 miles per gallon. Truck B costs $650 and gets 35 miles per gallon. If gasoline costs $4 per gallon, how many miles must Sally drive to make truck B the better buy?
   a. 500
   b. 7500
   c. 1750
   d. 4375

---

29. Given the equation $\frac{3}{y-5} = \frac{15}{y+4}$, what is the value of y?
   a. 45

   b. 54

   c. $\frac{29}{4}$

   d. $\frac{4}{29}$

The next two questions are based on the following information:

Joshua has to earn more than 92 points on the state test in order to qualify for an academic scholarship. Each question is worth 4 points, and the test has a total of 30 questions. Let x represent the number of test questions Joshua answers correctly.

30. Which of the following inequalities represents the scenario in which Joshua qualifies for an academic scholarship?
    a. $4x < 30$
    b $4x < 92$
    c. $4x > 30$
    d. $4x > 92$

31. What is the minimum number of test questions Joshua must answer correctly in order to qualify for an academic scholarship?
    a. 23
    b. 24
    c. 26
    d. 27

The next two questions are based on the following information:

Kyle bats third in the batting order for the Badgers baseball team. The table shows the number of hits that Kyle had in each of 7 consecutive games played during one week in July.

Day of Week	Number of Hits
Monday	1
Tuesday	2
Wednesday	3
Thursday	1
Friday	1
Saturday	4
Sunday	2

32. What is the mode of the numbers in the distribution shown in the table?
    a. 1
    b. 2
    c. 3
    d. 4

33. What is the mean of the numbers in the distribution shown in the table?
    a. 1
    b. 2
    c. 3
    d. 4

- 94 -

34. Given the data on the graph to the right, which statement best describes the rate of change?

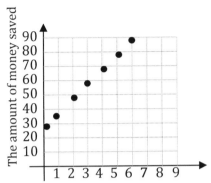

The number of days from now

   a. For every additional day, the amount saved increases by approximately one dollar.
   b. For every additional ten days, the amount saved increases by approximately one dollar.
   c. For every additional day, the amount saved increases by approximately ten dollars.
   d. None of the above

35. Elijah drove 45 miles to his job in an hour and ten minutes in the morning. On the way home in the evening, however, traffic was much heavier and the same trip took an hour and a half. What was his average speed in miles per hour for the round trip?
   a. 30
   b. $32\frac{1}{2}$
   c. $33\frac{3}{4}$
   d. 45

36. Given the sequence represented in the table below, where n represents the position of the term and a_n represents the value of the term, which of the following describes the relationship between the position number and the value of the term?

n	1	2	3	4	5	6
a_n	5	2	−1	−4	−7	−10

   a. Multiply n by 2 and subtract 4
   b. Multiply n by 2 and subtract 3
   c. Multiply n by −3 and add 8
   d. Multiply n by −4 and add 1

Science

DIRECTIONS: The science practice test you are about to take is multiple-choice with only one correct answer per question. Read each test item and circle your answer on the answer sheet below. When you have completed the practice test, you may check your answers with those on the answer key that follows the test.

Answer Sheet

1.	a	b	c	d		28.	a	b	c	d
2.	a	b	c	d		29.	a	b	c	d
3.	a	b	c	d		30.	a	b	c	d
4.	a	b	c	d		31.	a	b	c	d
5.	a	b	c	d		32.	a	b	c	d
6.	a	b	c	d		33.	a	b	c	d
7.	a	b	c	d		34.	a	b	c	d
8.	a	b	c	d		35.	a	b	c	d
9.	a	b	c	d		36.	a	b	c	d
10.	a	b	c	d		37.	a	b	c	d
11.	a	b	c	d		38.	a	b	c	d
12.	a	b	c	d		39.	a	b	c	d
13.	a	b	c	d		40.	a	b	c	d
14.	a	b	c	d		41.	a	b	c	d
15.	a	b	c	d		42.	a	b	c	d
16.	a	b	c	d		43.	a	b	c	d
17.	a	b	c	d		44.	a	b	c	d
18.	a	b	c	d		45.	a	b	c	d
19.	a	b	c	d		46.	a	b	c	d
20.	a	b	c	d		47.	a	b	c	d
21.	a	b	c	d		48.	a	b	c	d
22.	a	b	c	d		49.	a	b	c	d
23.	a	b	c	d		50.	a	b	c	d
24.	a	b	c	d		51.	a	b	c	d
25.	a	b	c	d		52.	a	b	c	d
26.	a	b	c	d		53.	a	b	c	d
27.	a	b	c	d						

1. A normal human sperm must contain:
    a. An X chromosome
    b. A Y chromosome
    c. 23 chromosomes
    d. B and C

2. During the process of oogenesis, primary oocytes produce:
    a. Sperm
    b. Eggs
    c. Oogonia
    d. Stem cells

3. In an oxidation reaction:
    a. An oxidizing agent gains electrons.
    b. An oxidizing agent loses electrons.
    c. A reducing agent gains electrons.
    d. reducing agent loses electrons.

4. The digestion of starch begins:
    a. In the mouth
    b. In the stomach
    c. In the pylorus
    d. In the duodenum

5. A neuron consists of three main parts. These are:
    a. Effector, cell body, axon
    b. Dendrites, axon, cell body
    c. Dendrites, axon, receptor
    d. Synapse, axon, cell body

6. Which of the following blood components is involved in blood clotting?
    a. Red blood cells
    b. Platelets
    c. White blood cells
    d. Leukocytes

7. A young woman fell and suffered a scaphoid fracture. Which of the following areas is the scaphoid located?
   a. Wrist
   b. Shoulder
   c. Spine
   d. Face

8. Name the valve that allows oxygenated blood flow from the left ventricle to the rest of the body?
   a. Aortic valve
   b. Mitral valve
   c. Pulmonic valve
   d. Tricuspid valve

9. Which of the following is considered an extensive property?
   a. weight
   b. density
   c. conductivity
   d. malleability

10. In the human skeleton, which of the following lists some of the vertebrae in descending order?
    a. Atlas, axis, thoracic, lumbar, sacral, coccyx
    b. Axis, sacral, coccyx, atlas, lumbar, thoracic
    c. Thoracic, sacral, lumbar, axis, coccyx, atlas
    d. Coccyx, lumbar, axis, sacral, thoracic, atlas

11. How does water affect the temperature of a living thing?
    a. Water increases temperature.
    b. Water keeps temperature stable.
    c. Water decreases temperature.
    d. Water does not affect temperature.

12. In which human body system do the white cell blood cells function?
    a. Respiratory
    b. Circulatory
    c. Lymphatic
    d. Endocrine

13. What kind of bond connects sugar and phosphate in DNA?
    a. hydrogen
    b. ionic
    c. covalent
    d. overt

14. What is correct about the hormones that stimulate male and female organs to produce male and female sex hormones?
    a. Female organs are stimulated by female hormones and male organs by male hormones.
    b. The same hormones that produce male or female sex characteristics stimulate the organs.
    c. The same hormones stimulate both male and female organs to produce sex hormones.
    d. The hypothalamus stimulates the pituitary gland's secretion of male and female hormones.

15. Which class of hormones is most likely to be released after a serious injury?
    a. Acetylcholine
    b. Oxytocin
    c. Luteinizing hormone
    d. Endorphins

16. Which of the following describes enlargement of an organ or tissue?
    a. Dystrophy
    b. Atrophy
    c. Hypertrophy
    d. Eutrophy

17. The triceps reflex:
    a. forces contraction of the triceps and extension of the arm
    b. forces contraction of the biceps, relaxation of the biceps, and arm extension
    c. causes the triceps to contract, causing the forearm to supinate and flex
    d. causes the triceps to relax and the upper arm to pronate and extend

18. Which structure of the nervous system carries action potential in the direction of a synapse?
    a. cell body
    b. axon
    c. neuron
    d. myelin

19. Which organ system is most responsible for maintaining control of body temperature?
    a. The skeletal system
    b. The circulatory system
    c. The immune system
    d. The muscular system

20. What is the function of an adipocyte?
   a. Fat storage
   b. Clotting
   c. Secretion of glucose
   d. Emulsification of fats

21. Examine the following reaction. Which of the answer choices is a possible set of products?

   ABC ----> _____

   a. 2AB + C
   b. AB + CD
   c. A + BC
   d. B + C

22. A particular individual has red hair and is six feet tall. Are these characteristics part of his genotype or phenotype?
   a. Hair color is part of the genotype; height is part of the phenotype.
   b. Hair color is part of the phenotype; height is part of the genotype.
   c. Both characteristics describe his genotype.
   d. Both characteristics describe his phenotype.

23. Which of the following lists best illustrates the idea of increasing levels of complexity?
   a. Cells, tissues, organelles, organs, systems
   b. Tissues, cells, organs, organelles, systems
   c. Organs, organelles, systems, cells, tissues
   d. Organelles, cells, tissues, organs, systems

24. Which type of nutrient is made up of amino acids?
   a. Carbohydrates
   b. Lipids
   c. Nucleic acids
   d. Proteins

25. Which of the following is not an example of a homeostatic mechanism?
   a. Shivering when the body temperature falls
   b. Increasing heart rate when blood pressure is low
   c. Weight gain when consuming excess calories
   d. Secreting insulin to decrease blood sugar concentration

26. Where is the scapula in relation to the olecranon?
    a. Distal
    b. Lateral
    c. Ventral
    d. Superior

27. When animals eat, insulin is released from the pancreas, stimulating glucose uptake by the liver. When glucose levels drop, the pancreas reduces insulin release. This is an example of which mechanism for maintaining homeostasis?
    a. Negative feedback
    b. Positive feedback
    c. Stress response
    d. Parasympathetic regulation

28. Which of the following is surgically altered during a vasectomy?
    a. Vas deferens
    b. Glans penis
    c. Prostate
    d. Urethra

29. The chemical equation below is unbalanced. When it is properly balanced, how many molecules of carbon dioxide (CO_2) are produced for each molecule of propane (C_3H_8) in the reaction?

$$C_3H_8 + O_2 \rightarrow CO_2 + H_2O$$

    a. One Half
    b. Two
    c. Three
    d. Five

30. What effect does a catalyst have on a chemical reaction?
    a. It speeds up the reaction.
    b. It slows down the reaction.
    c. It makes a reaction go in reverse.
    d. It prevents a reaction from taking place.

31. Where is the abdominopelvic cavity in relationship to the thoracic cavity?
    a. Dorsal
    b. Ventral
    c. Superior
    d. Inferior

32. Which organ system removes substances from the blood, combats disease, and maintains tissue fluid balance?
    a. Endocrine
    b. Lymphatic
    c. Nervous
    d. Integumentary

33. Which of the following statements best defines an organelle?
    a. Layer of polysaccharides outside the plasma membrane of cells
    b. Abnormal infectious proteins
    c. Specialized structures within a cell
    d. Collection of tissues used to serve a specific function

34. Which of these anatomical terms refers to the knee?
    a. Sternum
    b. Olecranon
    c. Patella
    d. Metatarsal

35. Homeostasis is defined as:
    a. Ability of human beings to keep body weight within normal limits
    b. Maintenance of a constant external temperature inside a room
    c. Ingestion of enough food to keep hunger pains from developing
    d. Tendency of the body to maintain a stable environment

36. A patient laying flat on their back is in which of the following positions?
    a. Prone
    b. Supine
    c. Lateral
    d. Medial

37. Which of the following is the result of bone marrow failure?
    a. Seizure
    b. Pancytopenia
    c. Paraplegia
    d. Pathologic fractures

38. Where would a nonpregnant patient with normal anatomy most commonly have pain in acute appendicitis?
    a. Right upper quadrant
    b. Left upper quadrant
    c. Right lower quadrant
    d. Left lower quadrant

39. Which of the following describes an experiment?
    a. The final math grades for a group of students passing through each year of elementary school are examined.
    b. The health trends of smokers in a small random sample are examined.
    c. Citizens in a local community are surveyed to determine concerns related to the next election.
    d. The effects of a new drug are tested on a group of participants.

40. Where is the gastrocnemius vein in relation to the femoral vein?
    a. Lateral
    b. Distal
    c. Superior
    d. Ventral

41. How many tissue layers does the uterus have?
    a. One
    b. Two
    c. Three
    d. Four

42. Which of the following causes varicose veins to occur?
    a. Atherosclerosis
    b. Incompetent valves
    c. Loss of skin turgor
    d. Loss of blood vessel elasticity

43. What is the process called in which a substance changes from a gas to a liquid?
    a. Condensation
    b. Evaporation
    c. Sublimation
    d. Vaporization

44. Which type of cells make up the myelin sheaths?
    a. Glial cells
    b. Dendrites
    c. Melanocytes
    d. Squamous cells

45. Which of the following steps comes first in a scientific investigation?
    a. Analysis of results
    b. Drawing conclusions
    c. Formation of hypothesis
    d. Performing the experiment

46. Which of these body parts does not contain melanin?
    a. Hair
    b. Nails
    c. Skin
    d. Iris

47. When a certain plant is introduced into an area, the population of a certain insect species declines. What can be concluded from this?
    a. The plant is toxic to the insect in question.
    b. The plant competes with and drives out plants that the insect feeds on.
    c. The insect population was declining anyway; the fact it happened when the plant was introduced is a coincidence.
    d. All of these explanations may be possible; further investigation is necessary to determine which is true.

48. What is the most important reason to formulate a hypothesis before conducting an experiment?
    a. It will increase the investigator's reputation and prestige if his hypothesis is proven correct.
    b. The hypothesis helps guide the investigation by suggesting what the investigator should be looking for.
    c. Formulating a hypothesis shows potential sources of funding that the investigator has given some thought to the experiment.
    d. The hypothesis directs which results to keep and publish; results that do not match the hypothesis should be discarded.

49. Which of the following techniques is most effective when defending a scientific argument?
    a. Citing other scientists who agree with your opinions.
    b. Showing the results of scientific experiments that support your argument.
    c. Describing your scientific credentials, education, and past accomplishments.
    d. Pointing out the fact that no one has come up with a proven alternative explanation.

50. Twenty people suffering from a disorder recover when given a particular drug. In order to verify that it was that drug that was responsible for their recovery, a hundred other people with this disorder are recruited into a clinical trial. Fifty subjects are given the drug, and fifty are given a placebo. Which of the following procedures would be most effective in testing whether the drug is responsible for their recovery?
   a. Ensure that neither the subjects nor the investigators know which subjects are given the drug and which are given the placebo.
   b. Ensure that the subjects do not know whether they are given the drug or the placebo, but the investigators are aware of who has received the medication.
   c. Ensure that the investigators do not know whether they are administering the drug or the placebo but the subjects do know which they are receiving.
   d. Ensure that both the investigators and the subjects have full knowledge of which subjects are getting the drug and which are getting a placebo.

51. When performing a research study, which of the following is NOT a good reason for using a computer?
   a. A computer can be used to store and sort large quantities of data.
   b. Computers can interface with instruments and record data efficiently.
   c. Using a computer eliminates all subjectivity and potential bias from an experiment.
   d. A computer can perform complex calculations more quickly and accurately than a human can.

52. An investigator wishes to test the effect of temperature on the durability of a certain material. He places five blocks of this material in a sunny area in a meadow, and five more in a cold area high in the mountains. He then monitors them over time. What is the main problem with this experiment?
   a. Ten subjects is far too small a number to get effective results.
   b. It is impossible to control for the fact that the blocks in the mountain were placed later.
   c. There are too many variables that are not being controlled for.
   d. Nothing is wrong with this experiment; this demonstrates good experimental procedure.

53. A scientist finds that the results of her experiment seem to contradict her hypothesis. What is the best course of action?
   a. Publish the results anyway, acknowledging that her hypothesis seems to have been incorrect.
   b. Keep trying the experiment until the results match her hypothesis.
   c. Publish the results, retroactively changing the hypothesis.
   d. None of the above; this cannot occur. The experimental results cannot contradict the hypothesis, by definition.

English and Language Usage

DIRECTIONS: The English and language usage practice test you are about to take is multiple-choice with only one correct answer per question. Read each test item and circle your answer on the answer sheet below. When you have completed the practice test, you may check your answers with those answers on the answer key that follows the test.

Answer Sheet

1.   a   b   c   d
2.   a   b   c   d
3.   a   b   c   d
4.   a   b   c   d
5.   a   b   c   d
6.   a   b   c   d
7.   a   b   c   d
8.   a   b   c   d
9.   a   b   c   d
10. a   b   c   d
11. a   b   c   d
12. a   b   c   d
13. a   b   c   d
14. a   b   c   d
15. a   b   c   d
16. a   b   c   d
17. a   b   c   d
18. a   b   c   d
19. a   b   c   d
20. a   b   c   d
21. a   b   c   d
22. a   b   c   d
23. a   b   c   d
24. a   b   c   d
25. a   b   c   d
26. a   b   c   d
27. a   b   c   d
28. a   b   c   d

1. Use of formal language would be LEAST essential when addressing which of the following audiences?
   a. a board of directors
   b. a grammar school class
   c. a gathering of college professors
   d. none of the above

2. Read the following introduction from an essay about Mary Shelley:

Mary Shelley conceived of Dr. Frankenstein and the hideous monster he created, which helped the English novelist to make an immeasurable impact on literature and popular culture.

Which of the following statements most effectively revises this introduction?
   a. English novelist Mary Shelley had an immeasurable impact on literature and popular culture when she conceived of Dr. Frankenstein and the hideous monster he created.
   b. Dr. Frankenstein created a hideous monster, and they were conceived by English novelist Mary Shelley, who had an immeasurable impact on literature and popular culture.
   c. English novelist Mary Shelley conceived of Dr. Frankenstein and the hideous monster he created and had an immeasurable impact on literature and popular culture.
   d. Novelist Mary Shelley from England had an immeasurable impact on literature and popular culture when she conceived of Dr. Frankenstein and the hideous monster he created.

3. Which of the following sentences contains proper capitalization?
   a. Last Summer, my family went on a trip to Niagara Falls in New York.
   b. Last summer, my family went on a trip to niagara falls in New York.
   c. Last summer, my family went on a trip to Niagara Falls in New York.
   d. Last Summer, my family went on a trip to Niagara Falls in new york.

4. Which version of the sentence does NOT contain any misspelled words?
   a. The suspect remained detained while the police conducted their inquisiton.
   b. The suspect remained detained while the police conducted their inquasition.
   c. The suspect remained detained while the police conducted their inquesition.
   d. The suspect remained detained while the police conducted their inquisition.

5. Which of the following versions of the sentence is written correctly?
   a. Because she wanted to reduce unnecessary waste, Cicily decided to have the television repaired instead of buying a new one.
   b. Cicily decided to have the television repaired because she wanted to reduce unnecessary waste instead of buying a new one.
   c. Cicily decided to have, because she wanted to reduce unnecessary waste, the television repaired instead of buying a new one.
   d. Because Cicily decided to have the television repaired instead of buying a new one she wanted to reduce unnecessary waste.

---

6. Which of the following answer choices is spelled correctly?
   a. intrude
   b. aclimate
   c. wisen
   d. alude

---

7. "We will depart as a class, but when we arrive we will split up into small groups." In this sentence, which part(s) is/are (a) prepositional phrase(s)?
   a. "as a class"
   b. "when we arrive"
   c. "into small groups"
   d. (a) and (c) but not (b)

---

8. Which of the following suffixes is NOT commonly used to form a noun from some other part of speech?
   a. -ation
   b. -ness
   c. -ity
   d. -id

---

9. I would like to go with you; however, I won't have time." In this sentence, what part of speech is the word "however?"
   a. Preposition
   b. Conjunction
   c. Conjunctive adverb
   d. Subordinating conjunction

---

10. "The tall man wearing a black raincoat, a yellow hat, and one red shoe entered the restaurant, walked to the back, and sat down alone at the smallest table farthest away from the staff and other patrons." This sentence has which of the following structures?
   a. Simple
   b. Complex
   c. Compound
   d. Compound-complex

11. "Although Ted had an impressive education, he had little experience working with individuals, which made him less effective at relating to them." Which kinds of clauses does this sentence contain?
   a. Two dependent clauses and one independent clause
   b. One dependent clause and two independent clauses
   c. Two independent clauses and no dependent clauses
   d. One dependent clause and one independent clause

12. Which of the following sentences is written correctly?
   a. Maya, my pet bird, can say "hello" in three languages.
   b. Jason, Peter Alice and Soojin all wanted to visit the new museum.
   c. Don't forget to bring your violin—music book—and music stand to the lessons.
   d. If you bring all of the supplies for the project I will provide the workspace.

13. Which of the following choices would be the best beginning for an essay on "Scientists Debate: Global Climate Change"?
   a. The Earth is heating up. The polar ice caps are melting and whole species are going extinct while governments and scientists argue over rules and regulations.
   b. The argument seems to be about whether climate change is really happening and if so, who causes it. Some scientists argue that people are causing the change.
   c. If the Earth heats up, what will our new world look like? Scientists who have dedicated their lives to understanding climate change have projected a series of scenarios that could happen.
   d. While few people can understand all of the issues related to climate change, one thing is sure: scientists do not agree. There seem to be several different views on how to look at climate change data.

14. Choose the sentence with the correct pronoun usage.
   a. "This mystery concerns my friend Watson and me."
   b. "This mystery concerns me and my friend Watson."
   c. "This mystery concerns my friend Watson and I."
   d. "This mystery concerns I and my friend Watson."

"Logan had already forgiven Marianne for telling his secret, and so when he was presented with a chance to treat her in kind, he simply did what he did best—he kept his mouth shut."

15. Which of the words in the sentence below is the past participle?
    a. telling
    b. forgiven
    c. and
    d. treat

---

(1) Throughout the song, he says, "Remember the better days."
(2) And he gives examples

16. What is the BEST way to combine sentence 1 and sentence 2?
    a. Throughout the song, he says "Remember the better days" and he gives examples.
    b. Throughout the song, he says, "Remember the better days," and he gives examples.
    c. Throughout the song he says Remember the better days, and he gives examples.
    d. Throughout the song he says Remember the better days and he gives examples.

This connection engendered an insatiable curiosity within Helen.

17. What does the word "engendered" mean as it is used in this sentence?
    a. Caused to exist
    b. Made sense of
    c. Connected
    d. Satisfied

---

18. Which of the following sentences is correct?
    a. The telescope accomplished amazing feats of enlargement, from showing the pock-marked face of the moon to the many moons of Saturn.
    b. The children all said that they had the best times of their life when they all lived together in the little two-bedroom bungalow.
    c. The study found that children frequently chose to use the entire bag of marshmallows for their hot cocoa.
    d. The astronomers found that the planets were following regular patterns and the philosophers argue about the nature of those paths.

---

19. The syllable –*tion* is a(n) _____ and turns a _____ into a _____.
    a. Suffix; verb; noun
    b. Affix; noun; pronoun
    c. Prefix; noun; verb
    d. Infix; noun; adjective

---

20. Based on the sentence contexts, which is true about the word *bark*?
    a. It is impossible to tell its meaning because its spelling and pronunciation are the same in both.
    b. The references to the dog in the first sentence and to the tree in the second define its meaning.
    c. "Bark" refers to a sound in the second sentence, and it refers to a plant covering in the first sentence.
    d. The meaning of this word is different in each sentence, but in one of them it is spelled wrong.

---

(1) The mechanic performed a number of diagnostic tests on the car.
(2) The mechanic used a computer to perform the diagnostic tests.

21. What is the BEST way to combine sentence 1 and sentence 2?
    a. While performing a number of diagnostic tests on the car, the mechanic used a computer to perform the tests.
    b. Although the mechanic used a computer, he performed a number of diagnostic tests on the car.
    c. Because he used a computer, the mechanic performed a number of diagnostic tests on the car.
    d. The mechanic used a computer to perform a number of diagnostic tests on the car.

The students' excitement about the beginning of summer vacation <u>pervaded</u> the whole classroom.

22. What does the underlined word in the following sentence mean?
    a. stood at attention
    b. spread throughout
    c. explained
    d. took note

---

23. Of the following, which version of the sentence is correct grammatically?
    a. I had seen her before, but yesterday was the first time I saw her indoors.
    b. I had saw her before, but yesterday was the first time I seen her indoors.
    c. I had seen her before, but yesterday was the first time I seen her indoors.
    d. I had saw her before, but yesterday was the first time I saw her indoors.

---

24. "Bess, who can draw beautifully, loves art; but Grace, who thinks very logically, prefers science." This is an example of which of the following sentence structures?
    a. Compound-complex
    b. Compound
    c. Complex
    d. Simple

When the chancellor would become <u>engrossed in</u> reading the day's intelligence, it was impossible for his subordinates to distract him with even the most important news.

25. Which of the following substitutions best captures the meaning of the underlined words?
    a. bothered by
    b. excited about
    c. occupied exclusively with
    d. confused by

---

(1) Because this the majority of survivors came from first class.
(2) They were able to reach the deck fastest to get a seat on a lifeboat.

26. What is the BEST way to revise and combine sentence 1 and sentence 2?
    a. Because, the majority of survivors came from first class as they were able to reach the deck fastest to get a seat on a lifeboat
    b. Because of this, the majority of survivors came from first class, as they were able to reach the deck fastest to get a seat on a lifeboat
    c. Because this, the majority of survivors came from first class, they were able to reach the deck fastest to get a seat on a lifeboat
    d. Because of this, the majority of survivors came from first class as they were able to reach the deck fastest to get a seat on a lifeboat

---

27. The words "aerobics" and "aeronautics" both have the prefix "aero" in common. What does "aero" mean?
    a. Light
    b. Speed
    c. Distance
    d. Air

The errors were becoming so frequent and <u>egregious</u> that the company had no choice but to force the humbled administrator into early retirement.

28. Which of the following substitutions best captures the meaning of the underlined word?
    a. thoughtless
    b. bizarre
    c. minor
    d. flagrant

Answers and Explanations #2

Reading Test

1. D. The point of the passage is to suggest that viewers should think more critically about assumptions and frameworks (such as the Western paradigm) that underlie the stories in movies they watch.

2. C. The author recommends that viewers think more critically about frameworks that underlie stories in movies; she argues that, if not, viewers may absorb biases with which they do not agree. An example the author gives of that bias is that it is hard to find a movie in which the hero is not supremely morally worthy. The author's identification of this as a bias implies that she thinks it is not the right choice. Her comment about the difficulty of finding a portrayal of an enemy that allows the enemy to be complex suggests that the author believes that more nuance and less absolutes would be an improvement in the U.S. storytelling of war.

3. C. The author said nothing about horseback riding.

4. A. The author suggests that these movies rarely show enemies of the U.S. to be complex or fighting for a legitimate cause.

5. A: The table reflects student scores for each quarter. The trend that can be seen in the graph is an increase in scores as the year progressed. The graph label mentions a test review, but there is not enough information about that to know if that is the reason for the scores changing.

6. C: The ad notes in the second sentence that candidates must be members of the California State Bar Association.

7. C: "Competitive salary" means on that is similar to the average offered for comparable jobs.

8. A: Since the ad suggests that candidates should be able to work in a self-directed capacity and as part of a team, it can be inferred that they might have both those work experiences.

9. B. The main idea of the passage is that the Food and Drug Administration (FDA) has a special program for regulating dietary supplements. This passage has a straightforward structure: The author introduces his subject in the first paragraph and uses the four succeeding paragraphs to elaborate. All of the other possible answers are true statements from the passage but cannot be considered the main idea. One way to approach questions about the main idea is to take sentences at random from the passage and see which answer choice they could potentially support. The main idea should be strengthened or supported by most of the details from the passage.

10. D. The passage never states that the Food and Drug Administration (FDA) ignores products after they enter the market. In fact, the entire fourth paragraph describes the steps taken by the FDA to regulate products once they are available for purchase. In some cases, questions of this type will contain answer choices that are directly contradictory. Here, for instance, answer choices A and B cannot be true if answer choice D is true. If there are at least two answer choices that contradict another answer choice, it is a safe bet that the contradicted answer choice cannot be correct. If you are at all uncertain about your logic, however, you should refer to the passage.

11. A. In the fifth paragraph, the word *deceptive* means "misleading." The root of the word *deceptive* is the same as for the words *deceive* and *deception*. Take a look at the context in which the word is used. The author states that the FDA prevents certain kinds of advertising. It would be somewhat redundant for the author to mean that the FDA prevents *illegal* advertising; this goes without saying. At the same time, it is unlikely that the FDA spends its time trying to prevent merely *irritating* advertising; the persistent presence of such advertising makes this answer choice inappropriate. Left with a choice between *malicious* and *misleading* advertising, it makes better sense to choose the latter, since being mean and nasty would be a bad technique for selling a product. It is common, however, for an advertiser to deliberately mislead the consumer.

12. C: Texting while driving is one of the key issues facing young people today: it's a fact that texting drivers have killed over 16,000 people between 2002 and 2007. While some people claim that any kind of distracted driving is dangerous, texting beats them all by keeping attention away from the road. This choice is the only one that takes a clear stand on the issue and provides a counterargument. The other choices are either too vague (A and D) or do not provide a counterargument.

13. C: All of these are good sources to use while developing a position on Civil Rights; nonetheless, first you must first familiarize yourself with an overview of the issue. A history textbook probably would be the most comprehensive and the least affected by personal opinion. Speeches, interviews, and blogs are great next steps in the research process, but these choices may prove too subjective to provide a necessary overview of the issue.

14. D: In the structural paragraph pattern of division (a), a whole is separated into its components by some principle (e.g., steps, body parts, etc.). In narration (b), the paragraph relates a story or part of one, e.g., an anecdote supporting its main idea. In definition (c), the paragraph defines a centrally important term in detail. In description (d), the writer uses specific details, including sensory, in the paragraph to show readers instead of telling them about someone or something.

15. B: Since the assignment is to read a biography, the librarian directs the student to the biography section of the library rather than to the Internet. She helps the student select a biography at his reading level. In this particular case, the student will benefit more from using the library's own resources than from using the Internet. The school library will probably have a biography of Thomas Jefferson, and the arrival date for the interlibrary loan would be too late for the student's needs.

16. D: This use of "smart" has a negative connotation: a "smart" answer here means a disrespectful or impertinent one. This is evident from the sentence context ("Eliot got into trouble"). (a) and (c) use the word "smart" with its literal denotation, meaning intelligent or competent. (b) uses "smart" with a positive connotation, meaning wise or judicious. The context "he got a good grade" informs this use: Eliot was smart to have studied, meaning he used good judgment when he prepared, evidenced by the positive outcome.

17. C: Sample 1's author cites evidence that is tangential to his argument; hence, it is not relevant. Sample 2's author cites anecdotal evidence which is inaccurate; hence, it is not factual. Sample 3's author cites evidence which is factual (accurate) and relevant (directly related), but not sufficient (an isolated example uncorroborated by any other sources). Criteria for evaluating evidence used in informational text include that the evidence be relevant, factual, and sufficient to accomplish the author's purpose (e.g., proving the author's point[s] and/or persuading the reader).

18. A. The word *deleterious* follows the word *delectation* closely enough in alphabetical arrangement that it is possible this word would appear on the following page. Answer choices B, C, and D are incorrect, because the words *dehydrate*, *delay*, and *deity* would all fall between the guide words *degressive* and *delectation*.

19. D: To evaluate source credibility, researchers consider not only an author's reputation in the field, but equally whether he or she cites sources (a). These two commonly (but not always) go hand in hand: generally, authors respected in their fields are responsible and cite sources. (In popular fields, some individuals gain favorable reputations without responsible scholarship. This is less common in rigorous academic fields.) In some rapidly changing fields, e.g., information technologies, sources must be current; in others, e.g., nineteenth-century American history (barring new historical discoveries), information published decades ago may still be accurate (b). Researchers must consider author point of view and purpose, which affect neutrality. Sources from certain points of view can be credible but may restrict subject treatment to one side of a debate (c). Audience values influence what they consider credible (d): younger readers accept internet sources more, academics value refereed journals, and local community residents may value mainstream sources such as *Newsweek* magazine.

20. C: The loss of coastal wetlands in Louisiana is an example of coastal island erosion caused by hurricanes, and so supports the statement. The other Choices are also statements that appear in the passage, but they do not provide direct support for the claim that many coastal islands are eroding.

21. D: The passage describes the loss of these coastal barrier lands to erosion. The fifth sentence then states, "the result is that recent hurricane seasons have been the most expensive on record." This establishes the cause-and-effect between barrier island erosion and monetary losses due to great storms.

22. B: The essay does not make comparisons or seek to define or persuade. Instead, this passage describes the role of coastal wetlands, gives examples of recent losses of these lands, and concludes these factors result in a substantial economic loss due to recent storms.

23. C: Based on the sentence that follows the one in which "mortal" appears, it can be inferred that this word is describing the president's wound as fatal: *The wound is mortal. The President has been insensible ever since it was inflicted, and is now dying.*

24. A: This article has eight headlines, each containing more specific information than the one that comes before. Though some of the information presented in the headlines is clearly opinion, the overall message that is being communicated is informational: Lincoln was shot at Ford's theater; he's still alive, but not expected to survive. An attempt was also made on Secretary Seward's life.

25. B: The notation at the beginning of the article lets the reader know that the information provided is an official communication from the government. There is no author indicated at the beginning of the article. This is something that is included in most newspaper articles. However, the article is written in the first person, and the identity of the author is revealed at the end:

I have seen Mr. Seward, but he and Frederick were both unconscious.

Edwin M. Stanton, Secretary of War.

Two of the answer choices reference people mentioned in the article. Finally, *The New York Times* is the publisher, not the author.

26. C: Answer C outlines the highlights of the article in the order they are discussed. Some of the other answer choices focus on certain points expressed in the article, but do not accurately reflect its overall message. Others present information that is not included in the article.

27. C: The first sentence expresses hope that the wounds inflicted upon Seward are not so severe that he would not be able to recover. The second sentence expresses the writer's fear that this hope may be misplaced, and it conveys that he is anxious about Seward's fate.

28. B: The first paragraph indicates that symptoms of magnesium deficiency rarely are observed, but a concern exists that people may have insufficient stores of this nutrient.

29. C: The passage describes both the causes of magnesium deficiency (dietary shortage or poor uptake exacerbated by gastrointestinal disorders) and its results (reduced functioning of the immune system and lessened resistance to cardiovascular disease).

30. B: According to the second paragraph, the kidneys usually limit magnesium excretion in the urine, but alcohol abuse and/or certain medications may affect this function. Impairment of this kidney function may lead to magnesium depletion. The passage does not state that magnesium uptake—a function of the intestines—is affected by alcohol.

31. B: The final paragraph indicates that magnesium deficiency can affect the absorption of "other cations," implying that magnesium itself is also a cation. The examples given, calcium and potassium, are also nutrients.

32. A: If a source is published in a peer-reviewed scholarly journal, or by a scientific publisher, professional society, or university press with peer review, a source is most often credible. Online publication does NOT mean a source is never credible (b): some are not, but many others are published in peer-reviewed scholarly journals. Author affiliations (c) with universities and institutions do inform online credibility. How many times a source has been cited in other sources also does (d).

33. D. The passage indicates that Gemma wants "to see as much as possible in a short period of time, while also giving herself a chance to relax and enjoy the experience." The book *The Top Ten: Beaches, Restaurants, and Sightseeing in Honolulu and on Oahu* fulfills this option most closely among the answer choices. Answer choice A limits the focus to waterfalls on two islands. Answer choice B focuses on a two-day hike. Answer choice C focuses only on restaurants, which will only help Gemma decide where to eat but will offer her no information about beaches and sightseeing.

34. A: It may be true that some businesses profit from buying up wetlands; however, the important point is that wetlands are disappearing. An ecologist noted that there are not enough private donors to buy these places.
This choice addresses the issue, uses information from both sources, but puts the emphasis on the qualified viewpoint (which is that of the ecologist; a physics professor may be smart, but ecology is not his field of expertise). Choice B puts the emphasis on the unqualified professional, Choice C

misinterprets the information provided by the expert, and Choice D does not address the issue, but addresses a side issue related to the problem.

35. C. Cora's interest in the boy band is clearly passionate. Her interest might have been *charming* up to a point, but given her parents' concern, it is no longer all that charming. While her interest might be *excessive*, that does more to describe her parents' response and does not represent a good synonym. Answer choice D, the word *covetous*, makes no sense.

36. A. The only dramatic increase indicated on the chart occurs between 1816 and 1921, when the Jewish population increases from fewer than 500,000 to more than 2,500,000. The population declined between 1939 and 1945, as well as between 1951 and 1960. There was a slight population increase between 1945 and 1946, but it cannot be described as dramatic.

37. B. From 1939, the Jewish population decreased steadily until the modern day, with the exception of a slight bump in population between 1945 and 1946. All other answer choices indicate a decline in population, and not an increase.

38. A. Chapter I of the cookbook contains recipes for breakfast breads, as well as muffins, so answer choice A is correct. All other answer choices reflect incorrect chapters of the book for these types of breads.

39. B. Chapter I of the cookbook contains recipes for biscuits, while Chapter III contains recipes for light soups. Answer choice A can only be described as half correct.

40. D. The announcement notes the following: "Students with more than one last name, or with a hyphenated last name, should use the first letter of the first last name for registration." Because of this, the only available registration option for Julie is on Tuesday, either from 1-3 PM or from 8-10 PM. Taking Julie's work schedule into account, she will only be able to register from 8-10 PM.

41. D: Answer choice (D) best summarizes the main topic discussed here. While choice (C) is a fact given about Tubman in the passage, it is not the main focus. Choices (A) and (B) are not discussed in the passage.

42. A: The author uses phrases like Tubman "was determined to gain her freedom" and "worried that she and the other slaves on the plantation were going to be sold" as he or she describes Tubman's life as a slave. The reader can deduce that author included these descriptions to illustrate why Harriet Tubman wanted to escape slavery, choice (A). The other answer choices are either insignificant details or not explained in the passage.

43. C: Clue words such as "as a child" and "later," as well as the use of dates, indicates that this passage is arranged in chronological order.

44. A: Paragraph 4 explains how Araminta Ross became known as Harriet Tubman. She married John Tubman and took his last name. She also changed her first name to her mother's name.

45. D. The only menu item that is vegetarian, with the possible inclusion of eggs or dairy, is the stuffed baked potato with vegetable soup. (In this case, the stuffed baked potato might have sour cream and cheese on it.) Answer choice A is questionable, particularly if the tofu takes the place of cheese in the lasagna; the question clearly states that Mirella prefers to consume eggs or dairy with every meal to ensure adequate protein intake. Answer choice B is incorrect, because Mirella avoids bread products. Answer choice C is incorrect, because Mirella does not eat fish.

46. D. Section 900 discusses history, so that is a safe starting point for Jensen. Section 100 focuses on philosophy, section 200 focuses on religion, and section 400 focuses on language.

47. D. Section 800 focuses on literature, and since Jensen is interested in the "written plays," this is the place to check for more information about Greek drama. Section 200 focuses on religion while section 600 focuses on science. Section 700 focuses on the arts, which could include theater as a performing art, but since the question specifically mentions Jensen's interest in written plays, answer choice C is incorrect.

48. B. Section 200 is the place to go for religion, so Jensen should check here for more about Greek polytheism. Section 100, about philosophy; section 300, about social sciences; and section 900, about literature, are not relevant.

49. A. The context of the sentence would suggest that Irmengard views her Aunt Fredericka's beliefs to be outdated. Answer choice B is itself confusing, as there is nothing in the sentence to suggest that Irmengard does not understand what her great-aunt means. Answer choice C does not fit the context, since Aunt Fredericka appears to disapprove of rather than be eager about dating and relationships. While Aunt Fredericka might be hostile to some elements of dating and relationships, the sentence does not indicate that she is hostile to the activities altogether.

50. A: Ask the student what his assignment is and what kind of books he is looking for. Before the librarian can effectively help the student, she must interview him about his needs. If his answer is vague, such as, "Well, I have to write this science paper," she should ask him a series of questions until she understands his exact need. Then, she can assist him in finding appropriate materials. Answer B assumes that the student knows what book he wants and does not know how to find it. This may not be the case. He may not know what book will help him. Answer C puts the problem off until another time, and the student may have a deadline to complete his assignment. Answer D takes valuable library time away from the student assigned help, and that student will not know as much as the librarian does about available materials.

51. A: Because the flu generally peaks as late as January, there is still opportunity to catch the disease. A flu vaccine is recommended. Choice 2 is incorrect; most people do not have the opportunity to avoid others for months at a time. The third response is also incorrect. There is no such thing as a double vaccine nor would waiting solve the issue of the current year. The local public health board has no jurisdiction over a private individual's choice of a vaccine, making choice 4 incorrect.

52. C: The passage explores the wide variety of self-improvement classes offered. As such, it touches upon the variety of content and subject matter, different venues in which the classes may be taught, and the range of enrollment sizes that may be encountered.

53. C: The passage points out that some of the subjects taught in informal courses may prove useful in the workplace and may make the student more desirable to potential employers. This includes topics such as computer science and foreign languages.

Mathematics Test

1. B. Multiply $120 by 24 months (a full two years) to get $2880. Add the thousand dollars for the down payment to get $3880. Find the difference between the entire amount all at once ($2600) and the amount paid in the plan ($3880). To find the difference, you subtract. The difference shows that $1280 more is paid with the financing plan.

2. C. $29 + r = 420$
$29 + r - 29 = 420 - 29$
$r = 391$

3. C. To solve, find the sum. $35\% + 4\% = 39\%$

4. C: One-fifth of $1,000 is $200; a donation of $30 per charity results in a total of $240 in donations. This amount is more than his allotted one-fifth of savings. Thus, the estimate is not reasonable.

5. B. Add to solve. The height of the window from the floor is not needed in this equation. It is extra information. You only need to add the heights of the two bookcases. Change the fractions so that they have a common denominator. After you add, simplify the fraction.

$$14\frac{1}{2} + 8\frac{3}{4}$$
$$= 14\frac{2}{4} + 8\frac{3}{4}$$
$$= 22\frac{5}{4}$$
$$= 23\frac{1}{4}$$

6. D: A circle graph is the data representation of choice, when wishing to compare percentages of a whole.

7. A: If x represents the number of hours of babysitting time, then the $2x$ represents $2 per hour and the $5x$ represents $5 per hour. So, the expression $12 + 2x$ represents Courtney's fee of $12 plus $2 per hour, and the expression $10 + 5x$ represents Kendra's fee of $10 plus $5 per hour. The equation which can be solved to determine the number of hours for which Courtney and Kendra charge the same amount is $12 + 2x = 10 + 5x$. Therefore, choice A is correct.

8. C: The circumference of a circle can be found by using the formula, $C = \pi d$. Since the radius is equal to 3 inches, the diameter is equal to 6 inches. Substituting a value of 6 inches for d and estimating pi to be 3, gives an approximate circumference of 18 inches.

9. A. Add the coefficients of the 'x-terms' together as follows: $5x + 4x = 9x$
Add the coefficients of the 'y-terms' as follows: $-2y + y = -y$
Put the x- and y-terms back into the same equation: $9x - y$.

10. B: The volume of a sphere may be calculated using the formula $V = \frac{4}{3}\pi r^3$, where r represents the radius. Substituting 3.5 for r gives $V = \frac{4}{3}\pi(3.5)^3$, which simplifies to $V \approx 179.6$.

11. B: The sequence can be converted to decimals and written as $0.875, 0.8, 0.5, -3, -8$. The hundredths place can be used to compare the first two decimals, while the tenths place can be used to compare all three decimals. The negative integers are smallest when the absolute value is greatest. Thus, the sequence for Choice B is written in order from greatest to least.

12. B. 410 ml × 4 containers = 1640 ml

Change to liters: $\frac{1640}{1000} = 1.64$

Add the liter that was already in the pot: 1.64 + 1 = 2.64 liters

13. C: Since the ratio of wages and benefits to other costs is 2:3, the amount of money spent on wages and benefits is $\frac{2}{5}$ of the business's total expenditure. $\frac{2}{5}$×$130,000 = $52,000.

14. D. Find the common denominator for the two fractions so that you can compare them. You can use the common denominator of 45, as follows:

$$\frac{2}{5} = \frac{18}{45} \text{ and } \frac{4}{9} = \frac{20}{45}$$

Look at the numerators: 18 and 20. The number halfway between them is 19, so the answer is $\frac{19}{45}$

15. C: If 1" represents 60 feet, 10" represents 600 ft, which is the same as 200 yards.

16. D: Thus, the expression can be rewritten as 4 + 12 ÷ 4 + 8×3. Next, multiplication and division must be computed as they appear from left to right in the expression. Thus, the expression can be further simplified as 4 + 3 + 24, which equals 31.

17. B: The amount she spends on rent and utilities is equal to 0.38(40,000), or $15,200, which is approximately $15,000.

18. C: If the exam has 30 questions, and the student answered C questions correctly and left B questions blank, then the number of questions the student answered incorrectly must be $30 - B - C$. He gets one point for each correct question, or $1 \times C = C$ points, and loses $\frac{1}{2}$ point for each incorrect question, or $\frac{1}{2}(30 - B - C)$ points. Therefore, one way to express his total score is $C - \frac{1}{2}(30 - B - C)$.

19. A: Percent increase is calculated with the formula $\frac{new\ value - original\ value}{original\ value} \times 100$. In this case, the percent change is calculated as $\frac{60.3 - 35.6}{35.6} \times 100 = 0.694 \times 100 = 69.4\%$. In Answer B, the percent change was incorrectly calculated by dividing the 2006 snowfall by the 2007 snowfall. In Answer C, the percent change formula was incorrectly set up as $\frac{new\ value - original\ value}{new\ value} \times 100$. In Answer D, the percent change was incorrectly calculated by subtracting the snowfall totals.

20. C. The total distance traveled was 8 + 3.6 = 11.6 miles. The first $\frac{1}{5}$ of a mile is charged at the higher rate. Since $\frac{1}{5}$ = 0.2, the remainder of the trip is 11.4 miles. Thus the fare for the distance traveled is computed as $5.50 + 5×11.4×$1.50 = $91. To this the charge for waiting time must be added, which is simply 9 x 20¢ = 180¢ = $1.80. Finally, add the two charges, $91 + $1.80 = $92.80.

21. C: The correct answer is 8. The total 20 + 13 = 33, but only 25 cars have been scored. Therefore, 33 – 25, or 8 cars must have had both a man and a woman inside.

22. B. First determine the proportion of students in Grade 5. Since the total number of students is 180, this proportion is $\frac{36}{180} = 0.2$, or 20%. Then determine the same proportion of the total prizes, which is 20% of twenty, or $0.2 \times 20 = 4$.

23. A: When plotting the sampling distribution of means, the distribution is approximately normal. As the number of random samples increases, the plotting of the means approaches a normal distribution.

24. C: The dilated triangle has dimensions equal to $\frac{3}{4}$ of the dimensions in the original triangle. Thus, the dimensions in the dilated triangle can be written as: $9 \times \frac{3}{4}$ cm, or 6.75 cm; $4 \times \frac{3}{4}$ cm, or 3 cm, and $7 \times \frac{3}{4}$ cm, or 5.25 cm.

25. A: Setting the cost of shipping equal to the amount received gives us the equation $3{,}000 + 100x = 400x$. Subtract $100x$ from both sides to get $3{,}000 = 300x$, then divide both sides by 300 to see that $x = 10$.

26. A. Each glass of lemonade costs 10¢, or $0.10, so that g glasses will cost $g \times \$0.10$. To this, add Bob's fixed cost of $45, giving the expression in A.

27. D: The area of the square is equal to $(30)^2$, or 900 square centimeters. The area of the circle is equal to $\pi(15)^2$, or approximately 707 square centimeters. The area of the shaded region is equal to the difference of the area of the square and the area of the circle, or $900 \text{ cm}^2 - 707 \text{ cm}^2$, which equals 193 cm². So the area of the shaded region is about 193 cm².

28. D. Let P_A equal the price of truck A and P_B that of truck B. Similarly let M_A and M_B represent the gas mileage obtained by each truck. The total cost of driving a truck n miles is

$$C = P + n \times \frac{\$4}{M}$$

To determine the break-even mileage, set the two cost equations equal to one another and solve for n:

$$P_A + n \times \frac{\$4}{M_A} = P_B + n \times \frac{\$4}{M_B}$$

$$n \times \frac{\$4}{M_A} - \frac{\$4}{M_B} = P_B - P_A$$

$$n = \frac{P_B - P_A}{\dfrac{\$4}{M_A} - \dfrac{\$4}{M_B}}$$

Plugging in the given values:

$$n = \frac{650-450}{\frac{4}{25} - \frac{4}{35}} = \frac{200}{\frac{28}{175} - \frac{20}{175}} = \frac{200}{\frac{8}{175}} = 4{,}375 \text{ miles.}$$

29. C. Rearranging the equation gives
$3(y + 4) = 15(y - 5)$, which is equivalent to
$15y - 3y = 12 + 75$, or
$12y = 87$, and solving for y,
$y = \frac{87}{12} = \frac{29}{4}$.

30. D: In order to qualify for an academic scholarship, Joshua must earn more than 92 points. Since each question is worth 4 points, and x represents the number of questions he answers correctly, the number of points he earns is $4x$. The number of points must be *more than* 92, so the inequality that represents Joshua qualifying for the academic scholarship is $4x > 92$.

31. B: Joshua must earn *more than* 92 points on the test in order to qualify for the scholarship. To solve this problem, determine the number of questions that he would need to answer correctly to earn *exactly* 92 points, and then round up (if the answer is *not* a whole number) or add one (if the answer is a whole number). Divide 92 by 4: $\frac{92}{4} = 23$. Joshua can earn exactly 92 points by answering 23 questions correctly, so he must answer more than 23 questions in order to qualify. Since the result was a whole number, add one to get the number of questions he must answer: $23 + 1 = 24$. Joshua must answer 24 questions correctly in order to qualify for the scholarship.

32. A. The mode is the number that appears most often in a set of data. If no item appears most often, then the data set has no mode. In this case, Kyle achieved one hit a total of three times, two hits twice, three hits once, and four hits once. One hit occurred the most times, therefore the mode of the data set is 1.

33. B. The mean, or average, is the sum of the numbers in a data set divided by the total number of items. This data set contains seven items, one for each day of the week. The total number of hits that Kyle had during the week is the sum of the numbers in the right-hand column, or 14. This gives: Mean $= \frac{14}{7} = 2$.

34. C: If a line is drawn through the points, for the horizontal change is 1, the vertical change is 10. The important thing is to notice that the scale of the y-axis has an interval of 10, so for every day, the amount increased by ten dollars.

35. C: To determine this, first determine the total distance of the round trip. This is twice the 45 miles of the one-way trip to work in the morning, or 90 miles. Then, to determine the total amount of time Elijah spent on the round trip, first convert his travel times into minutes. One hour and ten minutes equals 70 minutes, and an hour and a half equals 90 minutes. So, Elijah's total travel time was 70 + 90 = 160 minutes. Elijah's average speed can now be determined in miles per minute:

$$\text{Speed} = \frac{90 \text{ miles}}{160 \text{ min}} = 0.5625 \text{ miles per minute}$$

Finally, to convert this average speed to miles per hour, multiply by 60, since there are 60 minutes in an hour: Average speed (mph) = 60 × 0.5625 = 33.75 miles per hour.

36. C: The equation that represents the relationship between the position number, n, and the value of the term, a_n, is $a_n = -3n + 8$. Notice each n is multiplied by –3, with 8 added to that value. Substituting position number 1 for n gives $a_n = -3(1) + 8$, which equals 5. Substitution of the remaining position numbers does not provide a counterexample to this procedure.

Science Test

1. C. A normal sperm must contain one of each of the human chromosome pairs. There are 23 chromosome pairs in all. Twenty-two of these are *autosomal* chromosomes, which do not play a role in determining gender. The remaining pair consists of either two X chromosomes in the case of a female, or of an X and a Y chromosome in the case of a male. Therefore, a normal sperm cell will contain 22 autosomal chromosomes and either an X or a Y chromosome, but not both.

2. B. Oogenesis is the process that gives rise to the ovum, or egg, in mammals. The oocyte is the immature egg cell in the ovary. In humans, one oocyte matures during each menstrual cycle. It develops first into an intermediate form called the ootid, and eventually into an ovum. The prefix *oo-* is derived from Greek, and means "egg."

3. A. In an oxidation reaction, an oxidizing agent gains electrons from a reducing agent. By contributing electrons, the reducing agent reduces (makes more negative) the charge on the oxidizer. In the car battery, reduction of the positively-charged anode provides electrons, which then flow to the cathode, where an oxidation takes place. In an oxidation, an oxidizing agent increases (makes more positive) the charge on a reducer. In this way, the extra electrons in the negatively charged cathode are neutralized by the surrounding oxidizing agent.

4. A. The digestion of starch begins with its exposure to the enzyme amylase, which is present in the saliva. Amylase attacks the glycosidic bonds in starch, cleaving them to release sugars. This is the reason why some starchy foods may taste sweet if they are chewed extensively. Another form of amylase is produced by the pancreas, and continues the digestion of starches in the upper intestine. The di- and tri-saccharides, which are the initial products of this digestion, are eventually converted to glucose, a monosaccharide that is easily absorbed through the intestinal wall.

5. B. The cell body, containing the nucleus, is the control center of the cell and the site of its metabolic activity. Dendrites, which extend from this cell body, receive signals from other cells in the form of neurotransmitters. This triggers an electrical impulse, which travels down the axon to the next cell on the route of the signal. At the end of the axon, neurotransmitters are again released, cross the synapse, and act upon the following cell.

6. B: Platelets are cell fragments that are involved in blood clotting. Platelets are the site for the blood coagulation cascade. Its final steps are the formation of fibrinogen which, when cleaved, forms fibrin, the "skeleton" of the blood clot.

7. A: The scaphoid bone one of eight carpal bones that make up the wrist along with the radius and the ulna. The scaphoid bone is located at the base of the thumb. It is the most frequently injured bone in the wrist. The other carpal bones are trapezoid, trapezium, capitate, hamate, pisiform, triquetrum, and lunate.

8. A: The aortic valve allows oxygenated blood flow from the left ventricle to the rest of the body. The mitral valve allows oxygenated blood flow from the left atria to the left ventricle. The pulmonic valve opens to allow blood flow from the right ventricle to the pulmonary system. The tricuspid valve allows deoxygenated blood flow from the right atria to the right ventricle.

9. A. Extensive properties depend on the amount of matter present, while intensive properties do not depend on the amount of matter present. Density, conductivity, and malleability do not depend on the amount of matter present, and are therefore considered intensive properties. Weight and volume depend on the amount of matter present, and are therefore considered extensive properties.

10. A: From highest to lowest, the atlas is cervical vertebra 1, supporting the skull; the axis is cervical vertebra 2; next come cervical vertebrae 3 through 7, the bones in the back of the neck, which are omitted in all choices; then the 12 thoracic vertebrae are the upper back bones; below these are the 5 lumbar vertebrae in the lower back; the 5 sacral vertebrae (together, the sacrum) are the pelvic and hip-level back bones; and the coccyx or tailbone at the bottom of the spine contains 305 small bones, which are often fused together.

11. B. Water stabilizes the temperature of living things. The ability of warm-blooded animals, including human beings, to maintain a constant internal temperature is known as *homeostasis*. Homeostasis depends on the presence of water in the body. Water tends to minimize changes in temperature because it takes a while to heat up or cool down. When the human body gets warm, the blood vessels dilate and blood moves away from the torso and toward the extremities. When the body gets cold, blood concentrates in the torso. This is the reason why hands and feet tend to get especially cold in cold weather. The exam will require you to understand the basic processes of the human body.

12. C: White blood cells are known as lymphocytes, a clue to the fact that they function in the lymphatic system to produce antibodies and destroy virally affected or foreign cells. While they are also found within the circulatory (B) system, that is, in the bloodstream, they do not function there but are only in transit from the bone marrow to the lymphatic system. The endocrine (D) system includes the pancreas, male testes, female ovaries and uterus, and all of the body's glands, which secrete hormones regulating bodily function, metabolism, and growth.

13. C. The sugar and phosphate in DNA are connected by covalent bonds. A *covalent bond* is formed when atoms share electrons. It is very common for atoms to share pairs of electrons. An *ionic bond* is created when one or more electrons are transferred between atoms. *Ionic bonds*, also known as *electrovalent bonds*, are formed between ions with opposite charges. There is no such thing as an *overt bond* in chemistry. The exam will require you to understand and have some examples of these different types of bonds.

14. C: In both females and males, the brain's hypothalamus stimulates the pituitary gland to secrete luteinizing hormone (LH) and follicle-stimulating hormone (FSH). In females, these two hormones stimulate the ovaries to produce estrogen; in males, they stimulate the testes to produce testosterone. Hence, both female and male organs are stimulated by the same hormones, not each by female or male hormones (A). LH and FSH, the hormones that stimulate the male and female sexual organs, are not the same as estrogen and testosterone, which respectively stimulate the male and female organs to produce these sex hormones (B). The pituitary gland does not secrete these (D); it secretes LH and FSH.

15. D. Endorphins are a special group of neurotransmitters. When an injury occurs, endorphins are released, and are capable of reducing the severity of pain. They are also released during intense exercise and periods of intense relaxation. Acetylcholine (A), also a neurotransmitter, activates muscles and plays a role in attention and sensory perception. Oxytocin (B) plays a crucial role in female reproduction. Luteinizing hormone (C) plays an important role in female ovulation and testosterone production in males.

16. C: Hypertrophy is the enlargement of an organ or tissue. For example, benign prostatic hypertrophy (BPH) is the gradual enlargement of the prostate. It impinges on the bladder neck resulting in difficulty with voiding. It becomes more common as men age. Although it is a nuisance, it does not usually cause serious problems.

17. A: The triceps reflex forces the triceps to contract, which in turn extends the arm. Eliciting the deep tendon reflexes is an important indication of neural functioning. Without them, it can be a clue to serious spinal cord or other neurological injury. The physician should be notified immediately if a patient loses deep tendon reflexes.

18. B: *Axons* carry action potential in the direction of synapses. Axons are the long, fiberlike structures that carry information from neurons. Electrical impulses travel along the body of the axons, some of which are up to a foot long. A *neuron* is a type of cell that is responsible for sending information throughout the body. There are several types of neurons, including muscle neurons, which respond to instructions for movement; sensory neurons, which transmit information about the external world; and interneurons, which relay messages between neurons. *Myelin* is a fat that coats the nerves and ensures the accurate transmission of information in the nervous system.

19. B: The circulatory system carries blood throughout the body, and plays an important role in controlling body temperature. Capillaries below the skin contract or expand to release or contain body heat. Heat is also transported from hotter parts to colder parts to ensure an even body temperature. The skeletal system (A) protects organs and provides the body with its structure and shape. The immune system (C) helps fight off illnesses and infections. The muscular system (D) is what allows the body to move.

20. A: Adipocytes are primarily seen in adipose or fat tissue. Their primary function is the storage of fat. Adipocytes play a crucial role in maintaining proper energy balance, storing calories in the form of lipids, and mobilizing energy sources in response to stress.

21. C: A + BC. When the reactant ABC is decomposed, it will produce the products A + BC. The equation should read ABC --> A + BC. 2AB+C would not be a balanced equation according to the law of conservation of mass since this would produce 2A, 2B, and C. Since the original reactant was ABC, this could not be balanced. AB + CD is incorrect as the element D was not an original reactant. This does not follow the law that matter cannot be created nor destroyed. B + C has a similar problem as element A drops out of the equation. Because A was a part of the reactant, it needs to be part of the product.

22. D. An organism's genotype is its genetic makeup; its phenotype is the collection of its observable qualities and characteristics (each of which may be partly or wholly dependent on its genotype). Hair color and height both have a genetic basis, but they are not themselves genes. They are observable qualities, and are therefore part of the organism's phenotype.

23. D: An organelle is a specialized structure in a cell such as a ribosome. A tissue contains a large number of similar cells that perform the same function. Likewise, an organ is made up of similar tissues that perform the same function. Organ systems are two or more organs performing similar functions.

24. D. Proteins are essentially long strings of amino acids, joined end to end. There are twenty-two different amino acids that make up the proteins in the human body, and the exact sequence of amino acids determines what type of protein will be formed. This leads to a great variety of protein molecules of widely different shapes and purposes. Base pair triplets in nucleic acids (DNA and RNA) can represent amino acids to direct protein synthesis, but nucleic acids themselves are not composed of amino acids, nor are carbohydrates or lipids.

25. C: Homeostatic mechanisms are involuntary actions by organs, glands, tissues and cells to maintain balance within the body. For example, if a person becomes dehydrated the kidneys will retain fluid by decreasing urine output. Gaining weight when consuming excess calories (which is not involuntary) does not constitute an activity that is trying to help maintain balance for the body.

26. D: The scapula, or commonly known as the shoulder blade, is above the olecranon, commonly known as the elbow. Conversely, the olecranon is distal or inferior to the scapula.

27. A: Maintaining homeostasis means that conditions are kept stable and relatively constant. Negative feedback is a mechanism used to reverse or minimize changes in a system. In this example, negative feedback is used to keep the body's glucose and insulin levels stable. Positive feedback (B) is a mechanism that increases changes in a system. A stress response (C) describes the body's reaction to threats or pressures. Parasympathetic regulation (D) refers to activities of the nervous system, including slowing the heart rate and boosting intestinal activity.

28. A: The vas deferens from each testicle is clamped or cut. This prevents sperm from mixing with the semen that is ejaculated from the penis. The testes still produce sperm, but the sperm is reabsorbed by the body.

29. C. The equation as presented in the question is unbalanced, because there are unequal numbers of atoms of each element on the two sides of the arrow. The left side has three carbon atoms and the right only one, etc. To balance the equation, we need to add molecules of each substance so that there are an equal number of atoms of each element on each side. Consider each element individually, and add molecules to each side of the arrow so that their chemical equations balance. The complete balanced equation is as follows: $C_3H_8 + 5O_2 \rightarrow 3CO_2 + 4H_2O$
When balanced, there are three atoms of CO_2 for each atom of C_3H_8.

30. A. A catalyst is any substance that speeds up a chemical reaction. It may do so by any of a number of means: by binding to the reactants in a way that facilitates their reaction, by breaking them down into more reactive forms, etc. No matter how the specific catalyst functions, it lowers the activation energy of a reaction, resulting in a higher reaction rate. Enzymes are one example of a catalyst.

31. D: The abdominal cavity is inferior to the thoracic cavity, but superior to the abdominopelvic cavity. The thoracic or chest cavity is above or superior to the abdominopelvic cavity. The abdominopelvic cavity is distal or inferior to the thoracic cavity.

32. B: The lymphatic system is a complex network of lymphatic vessels and lymph nodes that run throughout the body. The lymph system is an important part of our immune system. It plays a role in fighting bacteria and destroying old or abnormal cells, such as cancer cells.

33. C: Organelles are specialized structures within a cell that serve a specific function. For example mitochondria supply energy to the cell by generating <u>adenosine triphosphate</u>. Ribosomes are the site for protein synthesis. The nucleus is in charge of all of the activities of the cell.

34. C: The patella is the medical term for the knee. The sternum is the bony structure that makes up the anterior chest wall. It is also known as the breastbone. The olecranon is the medical term for elbow. The metatarsals make up the bones of the midfoot.

35. D: Homeostatic mechanisms are involuntary actions by organs, glands, tissues and cells to maintain balance within the body. If a function is disrupted the body will readjust in an attempt to maintain balance. During periods of starvation the body will break down glucose reserves in order to maintain normal glucose levels.

36. B: The supine position is an anatomical position where a person is laying on their back facing upward. Prone is the opposite position. A person who is prone is on their abdomen lying face down. A patient is in the lateral position when they are lying on their side. Medial is not a body position; it describes being in the middle.

37. B: Pancytopenia is a result of bone marrow failure. Pancytopenia occurs when a person has a lower than normal number so white blood cells, red blood cells, and platelets. These three types of cells are all produced in the bone marrow.

38. C: In nonpregnant patients with normal anatomy, the appendix is adjacent to the ileocecal junction in the right lower quadrant of the abdomen. In atypical cases with abnormal anatomy appendicitis pain may be felt in the groin or the mid epigastrium. In pregnant patients the pain may occur in the epigastrium or even on the left side of the abdomen due to displacement of organs.

39. D: Only Choice D introduces an intervention to be studied. Thus, Choice D represents an experiment.

40. B: The gastrocnemius vein is found in the calf. The femoral vein is found in the proximal anterior thigh/pelvis. Since the gastrocnemius vein is found below the femoral vein it is distal or inferior to the femoral vessel.

41. C: The uterus has three layers. The inner layer is called the endometrium. The middle layer is called the myometrium. The outer layer of the uterus is called the serosa or perimetrium.

42. B: Incompetent valves allow backflow of blood causing the vein to become engorged. The engorged superficial veins become noticeable under the skin. Conditions such as pregnancy, genetic predisposition, and advanced age cause varicose veins to occur.

43. A. When a substance undergoes a phase transition from a gas to a liquid, this phenomenon is known as condensation. Evaporation and vaporization both describe the process of changing from a liquid to a gas, though vaporization is the more general term. Evaporation refers specifically to vaporization occurring at temperatures beneath the substance's boiling point. Sublimation refers to a change from a solid directly to a gas (as in the case of dry ice).

44. A: Glial cells comprise the myelin sheath, which acts as a fatty covering of nerve cells. Myelin sheaths serve to increase the speed of nerve signal transmission. Loss or damage to these sheaths lead to involuntary motor dysfunction such as those with multiple sclerosis.

45. C. After defining the question one wants to investigate and doing some preliminary research, the next step is to formulate a hypothesis. The researcher then tests the hypothesis by performing an appropriate and carefully designed experiment. The data gathered in the experiment is then analyzed, and based on the results, the investigator draws a conclusion about the hypothesis that was being studied.

46. B: Nails do not contain melanin. Melanin is the pigment that provides color to skin, hair, and eyes. Although the specific coloring or one's skin, hair, and eyes are genetically determined, environmental factors such as sun exposure can increase melanin production in the skin to help protect it from damage.

47. D. It's possible that the plant was toxic to the insects, or that it drove out another plant they fed on, or even that there was no connection between the introduction of the plant and the insects' decline. There may even be other possibilities beyond these. Based on this observation it's premature to make any conclusions about cause and effect. To determine which, if any, of these explanations is true, it would be necessary to conduct further investigations, including controlled experiments.

48. B. The most important reason to formulate a hypothesis before beginning an investigation is to focus the investigation by providing something specific to look for. In general, an effective experiment has a specific purpose and does not consist of just random manipulation of materials; the hypothesis actually defines that purpose. None of the other choices is a strong reason for formulating a hypothesis. In particular, choice D runs completely counter to good experimental procedure; an experiment that seems to disprove a hypothesis may have important implications, and should certainly not be cavalierly discarded.

49. B. The most effective way to defend a scientific argument and advance a position is to apply the scientific method: design and perform an experiment to test the hypothesis in question. If the results of the experiment seem to agree with the hypothesis, then this supports the argument, though further experiments may serve to strengthen it. While the other choices may have some psychological sway in moving people to agree with the arguer, they are not considered persuasive scientific evidence.

50. A. In clinical trials and similar investigations, the most effective experiments are "double blind", with neither the investigator nor the subject knowing who is in the treatment group and who is in control group. This is important in order to eliminate bias. If the subjects know they are being given a placebo, they may be more likely to not report any changes, or they may over report positive effects. If investigators know which subjects are given the placebo, they may inadvertently attach importance to subjects who are receiving the drug. Even if both the subjects and the investigators strive to be objective and not be swayed by their knowledge, the results may be biased unconsciously. Ensuring that neither the subjects nor the investigators know which subjects are the controls until the test is over prevents this bias from occurring.

51. C. Computers are useful in recording data from electrical instruments, in storing and analyzing large amounts of data, and in quickly and accurately performing calculations. However, the mere fact that one is using a computer does not automatically eliminate all possible sources of bias and subjectivity. A human still has to enter the data into a computer (or decide what data is to be recorded and kept, if the data is collected automatically), and to instruct the computer how to

- 128 -

analyze it. Even if a computer is performing the calculations, there are still many other stages in the experiment in which bias can creep in.

52. C. While more subjects may be desirable, there is no "magic number" that's correct, and ten may be enough to get useful results. It is not necessarily a problem that the blocks in the mountain were placed later, as long as this is taken into account in the analysis and he compares them against time after their placement. What is a problem, however, is that temperature is not the only variable that differs between the two experimental groups. For one thing, the air pressure will be different at the higher mountain altitude than it will be in the meadow. There may be other differences between the two areas that are not accounted for as well, such as wind and weather patterns.

53. A. A hypothesis is merely an educated guess as to what the investigator expects to happen. There is nothing wrong with finding out that one's hypothesis is incorrect. If the investigator already knew for sure that the hypothesis was correct, it wouldn't be a hypothesis, and there would be no need for the experiment. In fact, an unexpected result that contradicts one's hypothesis can often spark further lines of inquiry.

English and Language Test

1. B: Young people will respond to and better comprehend informal, friendly speech. However, you would not want to be too informal when addressing an educated gathering of college professors or a professional board of directors. Informal speech likely would weaken addresses made before such audiences.

2. A: This sentence offers the most effective revision. The syntax is clearer than the other answer choices. The writer achieves maximum impact by holding Mary Shelley's achievement, the creation of Dr. Frankenstein and his hideous monster in her novel Frankenstein, for the end of the sentence.

3. C: This is the best choice because summer is not a proper noun, but Niagara Falls and New York are proper nouns and require capitalization. A is not the best choice because summer is not a proper noun and should not be capitalized. B is not the best choice because Niagara Falls is a proper noun and should be capitalized. D is not the best choice because New York is a proper noun and should be capitalized.

4. D: Although the word inquisition means a prolonged process of questioning, it is not spelled with an <e>, as is question. The correct spelling uses an <i>, as in inquire.

5. A: The syntax of this sentence is correct. It uses a comma to offset the subordinate clause ("Because she wanted to reduce unnecessary waste") from the independent clause ("Cicily decided to have the television repaired instead of buying a new one"). Placing the independent clause, which is the most important idea in the sentence, at the end for emphasis also makes the sentence stronger.

6. A: Answer B should be "acclimate." Answer C should be "wizen." Answer D should be "allude."

7. D: Prepositional phrase "as a class" modifies verb "depart," with "as" meaning in the role of (a class). Prepositional phrase "into small groups" (c) modifies verb "split," with "into" meaning becoming or producing (small groups). (Note: Preposition "up" also modifies verb "split," creating the verb phrase "split up.") However, "when we arrive" (b) is not a prepositional phrase but an adverbial dependent clause, modifying the predicate "we will split" by specifying *when*, in the independent clause "we will split up into small groups."

8. D: The suffix –ation (a) commonly forms nouns from verbs, e.g., *converse* and *conversation, confront* and *confrontation, revoke* and *revocation, celebrate* and *celebration,* etc. The suffix –ness (b) commonly forms nouns from adjectives, e.g., *happy* and *happiness, kind* and *kindness, dark* and *darkness,* etc.; as does the suffix –ity (c), e.g., *formal* and *formality, sensitive* and *sensitivity, gay* and *gaiety,* etc. However, the suffix –id (d) commonly forms adjectives from nouns, e.g., *candor* and *candid, livor* and *livid, rabies* and *rabid, rigor* and *rigid,* etc.

9. C: *However* is a conjunctive adverb (adverb used like a conjunction) connecting independent clauses. A preposition (a) connects nouns, pronouns, noun phrases, and pronoun phrases to other words; in this sentence, *to* and *with* are prepositions. A conjunction (b) like *and, but, or, nor,* etc. connects words, phrases, and clauses. For example, in the rewritten sentence, "I would like to go with you, *but* I won't have time," *but* is a conjunction—specifically a coordinating conjunction, connecting independent clauses. A subordinating conjunction (d) introduces a dependent or subordinate clause, connecting it to an independent clause, e.g., "I cannot go with you *because* I won't have time."

10. A: Despite its length, this is a simple sentence—one independent clause, including a compound predicate (entered, walked, sat) modifying the subject (man) and a participial phrase (wearing) with multiple objects (raincoat, hat, shoe). All modifiers are adjectives (tall, black, yellow, red, smallest, other), adverbs (down, alone, farthest), prepositions (away from), prepositional phrases (to the back, at the smallest table, from the staff), and the participial phrase (wearing a black raincoat). It is not complex (b), having no dependent r subordinate clause; not compound (c), having only one independent clause; and not compound-complex (d), having only one independent and no dependent clause.

11. A: "Although Ted had an impressive education" is a dependent or subordinate clause, introduced by the subordinating conjunction "Although" and modifying the independent clause "he had little experience working with individuals." The second dependent clause is the relative clause "which made him less effective at relating to them," introduced by the relative pronoun "which" and modifying "he had little experience." Hence there is not just one dependent clause (b), (d), or none (c), nor are there two independent clauses (b), (c).

12. A: The other sentences either incorrectly use the comma (if at all) or the dash.

13. D: This is the best choice because it takes a look at the idea that scientists are not in complete agreement about climate change. Choice A takes only one position, option B is more of a detail that may go in the essay, and choice C is about a different topic.

14. A: "Me" is the object pronoun, and "Watson and me" is the correct word order. Just as you would say if you were alone, "This mystery concerns *me*," with another person added, you would say, "This mystery concerns Watson and me," not "Watson and I."

15. B: The past participle usually goes along with "have" or "had."

16. B: The reason that this is best is that this is the simplest way to express the idea in a grammatically correct sentence. A is incorrect because a comma is missing after *days*. C is incorrect because a comma is missing after *song*, and quotation marks are missing around the quotation, "Remember the better days." D is not correct. A comma is missing after *song* and after *days*, and quotation marks are missing around the quotation, "Remember the better days."

17. A: "This connection engendered an insatiable curiosity within Helen." The context of this sentence indicates that the connection Helen made between words and the objects they represent caused an insatiable curiosity to exist within Helen.

18. C: This choice shows the appropriate mood and tense. The other examples show mixed constructions (A) and errors in the construction (B) or verb tense (D).

19. A: *–Tion* is a suffix because it comes at the end of a word. It turns a verb into a noun: *attend* becomes *attention, convert* becomes *conversion, present-presentation, converse-conversation, ambulate-ambulation,* and more. Prefixes, suffixes, and infixes are all affixes. However, *-tion* does not turn nouns into pronouns (B). Pronouns are *I, me, we, us, you, he, she, they, them, it* (personal pronouns); *this, that, these, those, such* (demonstrative pronouns); *who, whom, which, that* (relative pronouns); *somebody, anybody, everybody, each, every, all, some, none, one* (indefinite pronouns); *myself, ourselves, yourself, himself, herself, themselves* (intensive or reflexive pronouns); and many more. The *–tion* suffix does not come at beginnings of words and hence is not a prefix, and does not make nouns into verbs (C)—such as *fright* into *frighten*—but vice versa. Infixes come in the middles of words, like *s* in *mothers-in-law* or *passers-by*; or in expressions like "abso-blooming-lutely" in *My Fair Lady*. *–Tion* is not an infix and does not make a noun into an adjective (D), such as *danger* into *dangerous*.

20. B: Because "his bark" refers to the dog in the first sentence, the context informs us that here "bark" means the vocal sound that a dog makes. Because "its bark" refers to the aspen tree in the second sentence, the context informs us that here "bark" means the covering of a tree trunk. Hence it is not true that it is impossible to tell the meaning in each sentence despite identical spelling and pronunciation (a). Answer (c) reverses the meanings in the two sentences. The word "bark" is not misspelled in either sentence (d). "Bark" in the first sentence and "bark" in the second sentence are both homonyms—i.e., they sound the same, and they are also homographs—i.e., they are spelled the same, but they have different meanings.

21. D: This choice makes it clear that the mechanic used the computer in order to perform the tests. Choice A makes the use of the computer appear incidental, while Choice C suggests that the mechanic was obliged to perform the tests because he used a computer.

22. B: "Pervade" means to spread throughout or to be found throughout something. The sentence tells the reader that the excitement did something in the classroom. Answer B is the only one that makes sense.

23. A: The past perfect tense of the verb "to see" is "had seen." The past tense of the verb is "saw." Thus "had saw" (b), (d) and "I seen" (b), (c) are both incorrect constructions. The present perfect tense also uses "seen," e.g., "I have seen her before." However, because the second clause is in the past tense, the first clause should be past perfect to reflect earlier times than yesterday. ("I <u>have</u> <u>seen</u> her before, but <u>today is</u> the first time I <u>see</u> her indoors" would be correct.)

24. A: This is an example of a compound-complex sentence, which combines two independent clauses with one or more dependent clauses. "Bess loves art" is an independent clause, modified by the dependent or subordinate relative clause "who can draw beautifully." "Grace prefers science" is a second independent clause, modified by a second dependent or subordinate relative clause "who thinks very logically." The two independent clauses are joined by the conjunction "but." A compound (b) sentence has two independent clauses but no dependent clauses. A complex (c) sentence has one independent and one dependent clause. A simple (d) sentence is one independent clause.

25. C: To engross is to capture one's attention utterly. To be occupied exclusively is another way of saying this. The other four emotions expressed do not contain the same implication of complete fixation.

26. B: It is correct because it is the simplest way to express the idea in a grammatically correct sentence. A is not correct. This sentence is not grammatically correct. C is not correct. This sentence is not grammatically correct. D is not correct. This sentence is not grammatically correct and needs a comma after class.

27. D: "Aero" is a Greek prefix that means "air." *Aerobics* is a form of exercise that causes an increase in oxygen intake and output; *Aeronautics* refers to the science of flight or aircraft.

28. D: Egregious means outstandingly bad or shocking. Flagrant means noticeable in a bad way so the two are the closest synonyms available. Thoughtless means selfish. Minor means insignificant. Bizarre means strange. None of these come close to the meaning of egregious.

49168094R00078

Made in the USA
Columbia, SC
17 January 2019